ILLICIT DRUGS

Recent Titles in
Health and Medical Issues Today

Stem Cells
Evelyn B. Kelly

Organ Transplantation
David Petechuk

Alternative Medicine
Christine A. Larson

Gene Therapy
Evelyn B. Kelly

Sports Medicine
Jennifer L. Minigh

Nutrition
Sharon Zoumbaris

HIV/AIDS
Kathy S. Stolley and John E. Glass

Medical Imaging
Harry LeVine, III

Medicare
Jennie Jacobs Kronenfeld

ILLICIT DRUGS

Richard E. Isralowitz and Peter L. Myers

Health and Medical Issues Today

GREENWOOD

AN IMPRINT OF ABC-CLIO, LLC
Santa Barbara, California • Denver, Colorado • Oxford, England

Library of Congress Cataloging-in-Publication Data

Isralowitz, Richard.
Illicit drugs / Richard E. Isralowitz and Peter L. Myers.
p. ; cm. — (Health and medical issues today)
Includes bibliographical references and index.
ISBN 978-0-313-36566-9 (alk. paper) — ISBN 978-0-313-36567-6 (ebook) 1. Drug abuse. 2. Drugs—Social aspects. 3. Drug control. I. Myers, Peter L. II. Title. III. Series: Health and medical issues today.
[DNLM: 1. Substance-Related Disorders. 2. Drug and Narcotic Control. 3. Public Policy. 4. Risk Factors. 5. Street Drugs. WM 270]

HV5801.I674 2011
362.29—dc22 2010040837

ISBN: 978-0-313-36566-9
EISBN: 978-0-313-36567-6

15 14 13 12 11 1 2 3 4 5

This book is also available on the World Wide Web as an eBook.
Visit www.abc-clio.com for details.

Greenwood
An Imprint of ABC-CLIO, LLC

ABC-CLIO, LLC
130 Cremona Drive, P.O. Box 1911
Santa Barbara, California 93116-1911

This book is printed on acid-free paper ∞

Manufactured in the United States of America

To all of my children, mother, and in
memory of my father.
—REI

To my children, grandson, and mother.
—PLM

Contents

Series Foreword

Every day, the public is bombarded with information on developments in medicine and health care. Whether the focus is on the latest techniques in treatments or research or concerns over public health threats, this information directly impacts the lives of people more than almost any other issue. Although there are many sources for understanding these topics—from Web sites and blogs to newspapers and magazines—students and ordinary citizens often need one resource that makes sense of the complex health and medical issues affecting their daily lives.

The *Health and Medical Issues Today* series provides just such a one-stop resource for obtaining a solid overview of the most controversial areas of health care today. Each volume addresses one topic and provides a balanced summary of what is known. These volumes provide an excellent first step for students and laypeople interested in understanding how health care works in our society today.

Each volume is broken into several sections to provide readers and researchers with easy access to the information they need:

- Part I provides overview chapters on background information—including chapters on such areas as the historical, scientific, medical, social, and legal issues involved—that a citizen needs to intelligently understand the topic.
- Part II provides capsule examinations of the most heated contemporary issues and debates, and analyzes in a balanced manner the viewpoints held by various advocates in the debates.

- Part III provides a selection of reference material, such as annotated primary source documents, a timeline of important events, and a directory of organizations that serve as the best next step in learning about the topic at hand.

The *Health and Medical Issues Today* series strives to provide readers with all the information needed to begin making sense of some of the most important debates going on in the world today. The series includes volumes on such topics as stem-cell research, obesity, gene therapy, alternative medicine, organ transplantation, mental health, and more.

Preface and Acknowledgments

Illicit drug use is a deeply imbedded characteristic of most societies. Its effects are shown in the form of illness, death, crime and violence, terrorism, police action and imprisonment, property confiscation, massive allocations of government resources, and many other ways of human suffering.

Worldwide, 200 million people, or 5 percent of the adult population, use illicit drugs—including marijuana, cocaine, heroin, amphetamines, and more—at least once a year. In spite of its connection to crime and terrorism, the production, trafficking, and consumption of illicit drugs continues to be a major international problem.

In the United States, the scope and impact of illicit drug use are profound. It is estimated that nearly 20 million people, or 8 percent of the adult population aged 12 years or older, are current (i.e., within the past month) illicit drug users. About 10 million people drive under the influence of illicit drugs annually. Among the 7.5 million persons, or 3 percent of the population, needing treatment for illicit drug use, nearly 80 percent do not receive it, and the main reason is that they do not have health coverage or cannot afford to pay for the cost. The United States has the highest incarceration rate in the world—one in every 131 U.S. residents—and a large percentage have illicit drug use problems and have violated drug laws and/or committed an offense while under the influence of drugs.

The economic impact of illicit drug use—including the cost of health care, social services, and criminal justice systems; losses due to crime, the costs of premature death and disability; and the amount spent on prevention, treatment and law enforcement—is enormous at more than $300 billion annually. Illicit drugs are a $60 billion per year industry, and to address its consequences, the U.S. government spends about $19 billion annually.

More than ever before, government and nongovernment policy and program decision makers, educators, service workers, and ordinary people are aware of the damage caused by the use of drugs. People are exposed to research, evaluation reports, policy proclamations and debates, and education. Many are aware that drug problems involve intervention with interrelated factors that include those of a health, judicial, educational, and welfare nature, and they also understand that there is no short-term fix. Although there is considerable investment of resources and effort to prevent and treat illicit drug use, problems shows no signs of abating. This complex issue has no simple solutions, and the challenges ahead are formidable. They include international control of illicit drugs from Afghanistan, Colombia, and Mexico among other countries; legislative actions and judicial decisions about the use of drugs like marijuana; policy making about prevention, treatment, and harm control; budget spending; and program support or elimination and more.

This book, *Illicit Drugs: A Reference Book,* examines illicit drug use from multiple perspectives. It defines terminology; reviews history; examines the scope of drug production, trafficking, and use in the United States, Europe, and elsewhere; describes the main illicit drugs of abuse; reviews the role of key people involved with the problem and how the problem has been and is being addressed; and lists sources of information that provide a direction for further inquiry. This book, we hope, serves its readers as an up-to-date source of usable knowledge about illicit drugs.

Acknowledgments

Appreciation is expressed to Sofia Borkin, MD, for her unwavering support of our efforts together. Gratitude is expressed to David Paige, Michelle Scott, other ABC-CLIO/Greenwood personnel, and the copyediting team for its helpful insight and suggestions that have moved this initiative forward through stages of preparation and production.

—REI

Appreciation is expressed to Susan Briggs Myers, LCSW, my muse and partner, and to my colleagues and friends in the International Coalition for Addiction Studies Education.

—PLM

PART I

Illicit Drug Use and Abuse

CHAPTER 1

Background

"Drugs destroy lives and communities, undermine sustainable human development and generate crime. Drugs affect all sectors of society in all countries; in particular, drug abuse affects the freedom and development of young people, the world's most valuable asset. Drugs are a grave threat to the health and well-being of all mankind, the independence of States, democracy, the stability of nations, the structure of all societies, and the dignity and hope of millions of people and their families" (United Nations 1998). Drugs are a problem in all nations that requires strategies and action to reduce the supply of and demand for illicit drugs; eliminate or significantly reduce illicit narcotic crops, including the coca bush, the cannabis plant, and the opium poppy; promote prevention, treatment, and rehabilitation opportunities; control the production of illicit drugs and the trafficking in arms involving terrorist groups, criminals, and transnational organized crime; persuade international financial institutions, such as the World Bank and the regional development banks, to include efforts against the world drug problem in their programs; and encourage communities, especially families, and their political, religious, educational, cultural, sports, business, and union leadership, nongovernmental organizations, and the media worldwide to work toward a society free of drug abuse (United Nations 1998).

Some success has been reported in containing the spread of the illicit drugs; however, there have been unintended consequences. For example, a criminal black market for illicit drugs continues to grow; public health, the first principle of drug control, receives only lip service and rhetoric compared with the attention given to public security; countries continue to supply illegal drugs despite considerable control efforts; drug abuse continues unabated and substances are easily obtained; and drug users, often unable to find treatment, tend to endure an life of stigma and marginalized status (UN Commission on Narcotic Drugs 2008).

Illicit drug use is a deeply imbedded characteristic of society associated with illness, death, crime and violence, police action and imprisonment, racial discrimination, inadequate and ineffective prevention and treatment interventions, children with parents who use drugs, property confiscation, as well as many ways of human suffering. Worldwide, it is estimated that about 5 percent of the total population ages 15–64 used illicit drugs at least once in 2008 (UNODC 2010); and, in the United States, 8 percent of the population aged 12 or older (SAMHSA 2009) are current (i.e., within the past 30 days) drug users. The problem of illicit drugs attracts more public concern and attention than any other social issue.

Key Terms and Definitions

When asked what a drug is, most people will say an illegal substance or a substance that causes addiction. But not every drug is illegal, and not every illicit drug causes addiction. The reason for the lack of a clear definition is that almost anything may be a drug. In the *Guide to Drug Abuse Research Terminology* published in 1982 by the National Institute on Drug Abuse in the United States, nearly three pages were used to define "drug," "drug dependence," "drug abuse," and "drug addiction" without providing a simple definition for any of them (Ray and Ksir 1990). What makes a substance a drug is not its chemical properties but how it is used by people. A typical example of this is the use and abuse of medications such as substituting methadone, a controlled opiate substance, for heroin, an abused opiate substance.

A drug may be defined as "any substance other than food that by its chemical nature affects the structure and function of the living organism" (National Commission on Marihuana and Drug Abuse 1973). A drug may be legal or illegal, harmful or helpful, as is the case of those substances used for promoting health. The meaning of a substance often varies with the context in which it is used—from country to country and over time in response to social and economic pressures. In the United States, for example, psychoactive substances like alcohol and tobacco were generally not regarded as drugs 30 years ago; today, the opposite is true. In general, laws exist covering most substances considered to be a drug. Indeed, there are international agreements among many countries that ban the use of certain substances except for medical and experimental research purposes. Such agreements, however, are subject to laws and means of enforcement that vary from country to country. Heroin, for example, may be used by those addicted to the drug for maintenance purposes in some countries but not in others. Cannabis oil may be used medically in the United States but not in many other countries; khat is legal in Yemen and cocaine in Peru and Bolivia. The use of alcohol is permitted in most countries, but not all—Saudi Arabia and other Muslim-dominated countries have very strict laws prohibiting its use. In most countries tobacco and alcohol are legal drugs. Cannabis (i.e., marijuana and hashish), heroin, cocaine, and methamphetamines are among the most commonly used illegal drugs in the United States.

From a positive perspective, a drug is used to maintain health, fight infection, reverse a disease process, and/or relieve symptoms of illness. In a neutral context, it is any substance that causes or creates significant psychological and/or physiological changes in the body. And from a negative perspective, it is often an illegal drug that causes addiction, habituation, or a marked change in psychological functioning.

Use

"Use" refers to the habits of those individuals who have tried or continue to use a drug but who are not dependent or addicted to it. The use of a drug is driven by one of two types of reasons. One group of people tends to use drugs just to feel good. They are seeking a good time and use drugs because their friends are doing it and they do not want to be left out. The second reason includes people who are suffering and use drugs to try to feel better or even normal. This group often includes people who live with poverty and/or who have been abused. It includes people with a variety of mental disorders like clinical depression, manic-depressive illness, panic disorders, and schizophrenia.

Many people use drugs to achieve a state of euphoria, pleasure, or relaxation, and it may be argued that they do not abuse the substances used. They tend to fall into different subgroups: (1) those who have tried a substance but have discontinued use, (2) those who use infrequently and primarily in response to social circumstances, and (3) those who use periodically but infrequently enough to avoid dependence or addictions (Leshner 2001).

Abuse

The American Medical Association once referred to "abuse" as the use of a drug outside a medical context. Used in this sense, abuse conveys the impression that a behavior is measurable, and announces to the world that the nonmedical taking of drugs is undesirable (Goode 1989). In 1973, the National Commission on Marihuana and Drug Abuse stated that the term "drug abuse" needed to be deleted from official pronouncements and public policy dialogue because it had no functional utility; it had become no more than an arbitrary, emotionally charged code word for drug use considered to be wrong. The term, however, is useful for differentiating users and abusers. Lorion and colleagues (1991) have stated that "users are those individuals who have tried or continue to use alcohol or other drugs but who are not dependent or addicted... abusers are heavily involved with drug use, while level of abuse may range from early dependence to life-threatening use, treatment is clearly the appropriate intervention."

Medical and government authorities have defined abuse as the non-medical use of a substance. This includes the use of prescription drugs in a manner inconsistent with accepted medical practices; the use of over-the-counter drugs contrary to labeling; or the use of any substance (e.g., inhalants, marijuana, heroin) for psychic effect, dependence, or suicide attempt.

The *Diagnostic and Statistical Manual of Mental Disorders, 4th edition* (*DSM-IV*), published by the American Psychiatric Association (2000), is the standard classification of mental disorders used by mental health professionals in the United States. The *DSM-IV-TR* states that drug use becomes abuse when it continues despite persistent or recurrent social, occupational, psychological, or physical problems caused by or made worse by this use. This maladaptive pattern leads to "clinically significant impairment or distress, as manifested by one (or more) of the following, occurring within a 12-month period." Among the diagnostic criteria are:

1. Recurrent substance use resulting in a failure to fulfill major role obligations at work, school, or home (e.g., repeated absences or poor work performance related to substance use; substance-related absences, suspensions, or expulsions from school; neglect of children or household)
2. Recurrent substance use in situations in which it is physically hazardous (e.g., driving an automobile or operating a machine when impaired by substance use)
3. Recurrent substance-related legal problems (e.g., arrests for substance-related disorderly conduct)
4. Continued substance use despite having persistent or recurrent social or interpersonal problems caused or exacerbated by the effects of the substance (e.g., arguments with spouse about consequences of intoxication, physical fights) (American Psychiatric Association 2000).

Dependence

Dependence involves compulsive and repetitive use of a drug, usually accompanied by craving, increased tolerance, and considerable impairment of health and social functioning. Among the diagnostic criteria of dependence are the following:

1. Tolerance, as defined by either of the following, increases: (a) a need for markedly increased amounts of the drug to achieve intoxication or the desired effect or (b) markedly diminished effect with continued use of the same amount of the substance.
2. The user experiences withdrawal, as manifested by either of the following: (a) the characteristic withdrawal syndrome for the drug or (b) the same (or a closely related) substance is taken to relieve or avoid withdrawal symptoms.
3. The drug is often taken in larger amounts or over a longer period than was intended.
4. There is a persistent desire or unsuccessful efforts to cut down or control drug use.
5. A great deal of time is spent in activities necessary to obtain the drug (e.g., visiting multiple doctors or driving long distances), use the drug (e.g., chain-smoking), or recover from its effects.
6. Important social, occupational, or recreational activities are given up or reduced because of drug use.
7. The drug use continues despite knowledge of having a persistent or recurrent physical or psychological problem that is likely to have been caused or exacerbated by the drug (e.g., current cocaine use despite recognition of cocaine-induced depression, or continued drinking despite recognition that an ulcer was made worse by alcohol consumption) (American Psychiatric Association 2000).

Types of Drugs

Drugs may be classified into five categories: (1) depressants (e.g., alcohol and tranquilizers); (2) hallucinogens (e.g., cannabis and LSD [lysergic acid diethylamide]); (3) narcotics (e.g., heroin and opium, from which morphine and codeine are derived); (4) stimulants (e.g., caffeine, nicotine, cocaine, amphetamines, and methamphetamines); and (5) other compounds (e.g., anabolic steroids and inhalants).

A more comprehensive classification comes from the *DSM-IV*, which lists 11 classes of pharmacological agents or drugs: alcohol; amphetamines or similar acting agents; caffeine; cannabis; cocaine; hallucinogens;

inhalants; nicotine; opiates; phencyclidine (PCP) or similar agents; and sedatives, hypnotics, and anxiolytics (i.e., drugs such as benzodiazepines that have an antianxiety effect and are used widely to relieve emotional tension). A 12th residual category covers everything else, such as anabolic steroids (substances like testosterone that increase muscle mass and strength) and nitrous oxide (American Psychiatric Association 2000). Following is a brief description of the classes of drugs.

Alcohol

Ethanol alcohol, not the isopropyl or methyl forms, is a drinkable liquid that can be addictive. The major types are distilled spirits (e.g., whiskey, vodka, and gin) and fermented beverages (e.g., beer and wine). Like heroin, cocaine, and LSD, alcohol is a psychoactive substance. It is a central nervous system depressant that affects brain function, lowers inhibitions, and impairs judgment, coordination, reflexes, vision, and memory. It may cause blackouts, damage every organ in the body, and increase the risk of life-threatening diseases, including cancer. Drinking can lead to risky behaviors including unprotected sex that may expose a person to human immunodeficiency virus/acquired immunodeficiency syndrome (HIV/AIDS) and other sexually transmitted diseases or cause unwanted pregnancy.

Amphetamines

Amphetamines are drugs that stimulate the central nervous system producing an increased state of arousal, sense of confidence, and euphoria. Users tend to be in a state of hyperactivity, agitation, or exhaustion. Prolonged use of amphetamines can cause irrational and paranoid behavior. These substances are used to treat such problems as depression, obesity, attention disorders, and narcolepsy. Most nonmedically prescribed amphetamines, however, are produced in clandestine laboratories and sold illegally. Presently, two substances tend to define this category of substances—methamphetamine and ecstasy.

Methamphetamine (or "meth"), a synthetic stimulant that is also known as crank, crystal, crystal meth, and speed, has been the most prevalent clandestinely produced controlled substance in the United States since 1979. Meth is made with relatively low-cost materials; it is an odorless, bitter-tasting, white crystalline powder that dissolves in water or alcohol. It is a powerfully addictive substance that affects the brain and the rest of the central nervous system. The active ingredient is ephedrine or pseudoephedrine—a common ingredient found in prescribed or over-the-counter medicines. Methamphetamine in powder form is smoked, snorted, or injected intravenously. Crystal meth or "ice" is a concentrated form of methamphetamine that resembles tiny chunks of translucent glass. As crack is to cocaine, ice is to methamphetamine. The effects of methamphetamine last 6 to 8 hours depending on the way it is used.

Ecstasy (3,4-methylenedioxymethamphetamine or MDMA) is a synthetic, psychoactive substance with stimulant and mild hallucinogenic properties; it is often used in pill form. It was patented in 1913 by the German pharmaceutical company Merck. The substance is structurally similar to methamphetamine and the hallucinogen mescaline. Ecstasy has been associated with verbal memory impairments and poorer memory performance, and it may affect the user's ability to reason verbally or sustain attention. Ecstasy is used in social settings such as nightclubs and dance clubs, private homes, college dormitories, and bars. The drug combines two opposite effects, stimulation and relaxation. The effects are similar, though more intense, to the popular antidepressant fluoxetine (e.g., Prozac and Sarafem). It is often used in combination with other drugs—mostly alcohol, but also with other club drugs like GHB (gamma-hydroxybutyric acid), ketamine, marijuana, methamphetamine, psilocybin mushrooms, and LSD. Ecstasy has been used for therapeutic purposes to treat anxiety and depression among cancer patients and post-traumatic stress disorder.

Caffeine

Caffeine, one of the oldest stimulants known, affects the central nervous system. It is a mildly addictive, naturally occurring substance found in plants like cocoa beans, tea leaves, and kola nuts. It is present in coffee, tea, soft drinks, and over-the-counter drugs such as NoDoz, Anacin, and Excedrin. In one form or another, it is consumed by 90 percent of the people in the world without any serious health problems. Coffee, brewed from the coffee bean, is the main source of caffeine. Caffeine content in coffee varies widely depending on the type of coffee bean used and how coffee is prepared. In general, the amount of caffeine in one cup of drip coffee ranges from 40 milligrams to about 100 milligrams. Generally, dark-roast coffee has less caffeine than lighter roasts because the roasting process reduces the bean's caffeine content. The caffeine ingested by drinking as many as four cups of coffee a day is not harmful for most people. However, excess caffeine can produce a range of unpleasant side effects, including restlessness, anxiousness, irritability, and headache. Additionally, serious side effects may occur, including convulsions, difficulty breathing, light flashes, vomiting, diarrhea, ringing ears, and abnormal heart rhythms. A person who stops using caffeine may experience withdrawal symptoms (NIH 2008). The symptoms of caffeine overdose (caffeinism) will vary according to individual differences and the amount consumed. Energy drinks like Red Bull have a caffeine level equivalent to a cup of coffee, and the caffeine content of soft drinks may vary: Mountain Dew and Pepsi One contain 55 milligrams in a 12-ounce serving and Coca-Cola Classic contains 34 milligrams in a 12-ounce serving (Erowid 2009).

Cannabis (Marijuana and Hashish)

"Cannabis is a leafy plant which grows wild in many areas of the world. It is cultivated both indoors and out for the production of its flowering tops. The most commonly used form of cannabis are the leaves and flowering tops (buds) that may be either smoked or eaten; it also comes in a more concentrated resinous form called hashish, and as a sticky black liquid called hash oil" (Erowid 2009). Marijuana is the most commonly used illegal substance; it is also known as cannabis, pot, weed, ganja, among other names. Although 60 cannabinoids (certain chemical compounds) are found in marijuana, the psychoactive one that most affects the brain is THC (delta-9-tetrahydrocannabinol). The THC level in marijuana has increased over the past quarter century from less than 1 percent to as much as 17 percent; the current average amount from seized samples is 10.1 percent compared with just under 4 percent reported in 1983 (ONDCP 2009). Use of the substance is a criminal offense under U.S. federal law. Local and state enforcement of marijuana violations vary from location to location. From a medical perspective, marijuana has been found to be beneficial in treating the symptoms of AIDS, cancer, multiple sclerosis, glaucoma, and other serious conditions.

Cocaine

Cocaine is a powerfully addictive stimulant drug extracted and refined from the coca plant, which is grown primarily in the Andean region of South America. It is sold on the street as a fine, white powder that is most often snorted. The two forms of cocaine are hydrochloride salt and freebase. The salt dissolves in water, and in a liquid form it can be injected with a needle or sprayed in the nose. The freebase form can be smoked. Crack is the street name of a smokable form of cocaine. The term "crack" refers to the crackling sound heard when it is heated. Crack vaporizes at smoking temperatures, which provides more effect with less substance; that is, it provides a faster onset and a more intense high than powder cocaine. No matter how cocaine is taken, it is dangerous. People who use cocaine often do not eat or sleep regularly and experience an increased heart rate, muscle spasms, convulsions, and respiratory and digestive problems.

Hallucinogens

Hallucinogenic drugs are substances that distort the perception of objective reality—including direction, distance, and time. "These drugs can produce unpredictable, erratic and violent behavior in users that sometimes leads to serious injuries and death" (SAMHSA 2009). In the past, plants and fungi that contained hallucinogenic substances were abused. Currently, these hallucinogenic substances are produced synthetically to provide a higher potency. Among the well-known hallucinogens is phencyclidine, otherwise known as PCP, angel dust, or love boat. This substance, described as a separate category in *DSM–IV* (see the PCP section further on in this chapter), can be snorted, smoked, eaten, or injected, and because it is fat soluble, it takes a prolonged period to leave the body (McCann et al. 1994). Though LSD is a powerful synthesized psychoactive substance, its use is unlikely to cause addiction in most people, and there is no physical addiction or withdrawal; however, it can become psychologically habit forming. Other substances in this category are peyote—a small, button-shaped cactus that is dried and eaten—and San Pedro, a cactus. The effects of these plants come from its main active alkaloid, mescaline. Dextromethorphan (sometimes called "DXM" or "robo") is an ingredient in many over-the-counter cold and cough medications, and it is considered safe and effective at the doses recommended for treating coughs. However, dextromethorphan may produce dissociative effects similar to those of PCP and ketamine, a substance used as a veterinary and human anesthetic, when taken at higher doses.

Inhalants

Inhalants are breathable chemical gases abused to produce psychoactive effects. Among the substances abused as inhalants are solvents such as gasoline, glues, and nail polish remover; the gases used as propellants in butane lighters; aerosols, including spray paints and hair spray; refrigerants; and even the volatile nitrates found in room deodorizers. Inhalants affect the brain with great speed and force, and because of this, they are capable of causing irreversible physical and mental damage. Young children and adolescents are among those most likely to abuse inhalants—in fact, among eighth graders, inhalants are the most commonly tried of all illicit drugs. Nitrites are a special class of inhalants used primarily as sexual enhancers. Chronic inhalant users may exhibit signs such as anxiety, excitability, irritability, or restlessness.

> Sniffing highly concentrated amounts of the chemicals in solvents or aerosol sprays can directly induce heart failure and death within minutes of a session of repeated inhalations. This syndrome, known as "sudden sniffing

> death," can result from a single session of inhalant use by an otherwise healthy young person. Sudden sniffing death is particularly associated with the abuse of butane, propane, and chemicals in aerosols. High concentrations of inhalants may also cause death from suffocation by displacing oxygen in the lungs, even when using aerosols or volatile products for their legitimate purposes (i.e., painting, cleaning), it is wise to do so in a well-ventilated room or outdoors. (NIDA 2009)

Nicotine

Nicotine is the drug in tobacco that causes addiction. The substance is found in cigarettes, cigars, pipe tobacco, and smokeless tobacco products such as snuff and chewing tobacco. In the form of smoking, the substance is the most common cause of lung cancer and preventable death in the United States. The pharmacological and biological processes that determine tobacco addiction are similar to those that determine addiction to drugs such as heroin and cocaine. Nicotine can act as both a stimulant and a sedative. Chronic exposure to nicotine results in addiction. Tolerance, the condition in which higher doses of a drug are required to produce the same initial stimulation, results from repeated exposure to nicotine. The withdrawal syndrome associated with cessation of nicotine use includes unpleasant symptoms that can last for a month or more and typically drive people back to tobacco use. Most nicotine users who try to quit without seeking treatment relapse within one week and more than 90 percent fail. Women who smoke during pregnancy are at greater risk than nonsmokers for premature delivery, and there is a risk of lower birth weight for infants carried to term. Among the risks associated with nicotine use, especially in the form of smoking, are decreased senses of smell and taste; frequent colds; bleeding gums and frequent mouth sores; wheezing and coughing; bad breath; yellow-stained teeth and fingers; gastric ulcers; chronic bronchitis; increase in heart rate and blood pressure; emphysema; heart disease; stroke; and cancer of the mouth, larynx, pharynx, esophagus, lungs, pancreas, cervix, uterus, and bladder (NIDA 1998).

Opiates

Opiates, referred to as narcotics, are a group of drugs that include opium, morphine, heroin, and codeine. Opium appears as dark brown chunks or as a powder and is usually smoked or eaten. Afghanistan is the world's largest provider of opium. Heroin can be a white or brownish powder that is usually dissolved in water and then injected. "The differences in color are due to impurities left from the manufacturing process or the presence of additives. Another form of heroin, 'black tar' heroin, is primarily available in the western and southwestern United States. This heroin, which is produced in Mexico, may be sticky like roofing tar or hard like coal, with its color varying from dark brown to black" (ONDCP 2010). Other opiates come in a variety of forms, including capsules (e.g., oxycodone), tablets, syrups, solutions, and suppositories. The substances may be eaten, but they are generally smoked, sniffed, or injected subcutaneously or intravenously. Subcutaneous injection, referred to as "skin-popping," produces a slower absorption, a lower degree of euphoria, but longer-lasting effects, including characteristic marks on the skin. Injection is the most efficient way to administer low-purity heroin. The availability of high-purity heroin, however, and the fear of infection by sharing needles have made snorting and smoking the more common methods of ingesting the drug. Prescription opiates, as well as illegal opiates like heroin, become morphine when they hit the brain, producing a calming, dreamy effect that blocks pain. People under the influence of opiates appear calm or sometimes sleepy, and they have a tendency to take everything in stride. Pure opiates cause relatively little body damage; however, substances sold on the streets as opiates usually contain a large amount of contaminants, including poison that can produce serious damage or even death to the user. Unlike stimulants, opiates do not produce a psychotic state when used in its pure form and have the ability to reduce or eliminate psychotic symptoms in mental patients.

PCP

PCP is a synthetic substance that was developed in the 1950 as an intravenous anesthetic. Virtually all PCP encountered in the United States is produced in clandestine laboratories. "In its pure form, PCP is a white crystalline powder that readily dissolves in water; however, most PCP on the street contains a number of contaminates causing the color to range from tan to brown, with a consistency ranging from powder to a gummy mass" (DEA 2010). PCP is most commonly sold as a powder or liquid, but it may come in tablet or capsule form. The substance affects the user at different times as a stimulant, hallucinogen, analgesic, or sedative. It can be snorted, smoked, or swallowed. For smoking, PCP is often applied to a leafy material such as marijuana, cigar tobacco, mint, parsley, or oregano. Among the names given for the substance are "angel dust," "wack," and "rocket fuel." PCP is addictive and leads to psychological dependence, craving, and compulsive PCP-seeking behavior. Its use is associated with a number of risks and many believe it to be one of the most dangerous drugs of abuse. Among the physical consequences are numbness, slurred speech, loss of coordination, rapid and involuntary eye movements, auditory hallucinations, image distortion, severe mood disorders, and amnesia. In some people PCP use may result in acute anxiety, a feeling of impending doom, paranoia, and violent hostility. Sometimes it produces a psychosis indistinguishable from schizophrenia, and nausea, drooling, dizziness, and memory loss have been reported as well.

Sedatives, Hypnotics, and Anxiolytics

This class of drugs when abused is commonly known as "downers." They include prescription drugs used to reduce anxiety or facilitate sleep. The most commonly abused drugs in this class are the benzodiazepines (Valium, Xanax, Ativan, Halcion, and others) and barbiturates (phenobarbital, Seconal, Nembutal, and Amytal). Other substances in this category, such as GHB, flunitrazepam (Rohypnol), and ketamine, are known as date rape or club drugs, because they are sedatives that affect judgment and behavior and can put a person at risk for unwanted or risky sexual activity. GHB is a central nervous system depressant usually sold as an odorless, colorless liquid in spring water bottles or as a powder and mixed with beverages. In addition to being used in drug-assisted rapes, GHB is used as a muscle-stimulating growth hormone, sleep aid, and aphrodisiac. This substance, smuggled into the United States primarily from Mexico because it is no longer sold in the country, is used mostly with beer as an alcohol extender and disinhibitory agent. Ketamine, a white powder, can cause hallucinations, distortions, a feeling of being out of control, and memory loss, among other problems.

References

American Psychiatric Association. 2000. *Diagnostic and Statistical Manual of Mental Disorders*, 4th ed. (text revision). Washington, DC: American Psychiatric Association.

Drug Enforcement Agency (DEA). 2010. "Phencyclidine (PCP)." Available at: http://www.usdoj.gov/dea/concern/pcp.html. Accessed February 23, 2010.

Erowid. 2008. "Caffeine." Available at: http://www.erowid.org/chemicals/caffeine. Accessed May 4, 2009.

Erowid. 2009. "Cannabis." Available at: http://www.erowid.org/plants/cannabis/cannabis_basics.shtml. Accessed May 4, 2009.

Goode, E. 1989. *Drugs in American Society.* New York: McGraw-Hill.

Leshner, A. 2001. *Why Do Sally and Johnny Use Drugs?* Available at: http://archives.drugabuse.gov/Published_Articles/Sally.html. Accessed September 1, 2010.

Lorion R., D. Bussell, and R. Goldberg. 1991. "Identification of Youth at High Risk for Alcohol or Other Drug Problems." In *Preventing Adolescent Drug Use: From Theory to Practice*, ed. E. Goplerud, 53–90. OSAP, DHHS

Pub. No. (ADM) 91–1725. Washington, DC: U.S. Government Printing Office.

McCann, M., R. Rawson, J. Obert, and A. Hasson. 1994. *Treatment of Opiate Addiction with Methadone*. Rockville, Md.: U.S. Department of Health and Human Services.

National Commission on Marijuana and Drug Abuse. 1973. *Drug Use in America: Problem in Perspective.* Available at: http://www.drugtext.org/index.php/en/reports/233-the-report-of-the-national-commission-on-marihuana-and-drug-abuse. Accessed July 4, 2009.

National Institute on Drug Abuse (NIDA). 1998. "NIDA Notes—Facts about Nicotine and Tobacco Products." Available at: http://archives.drugabuse.gov/NIDA_Notes/NNVol13N3/tearoff.html. Accessed September 3, 2010.

National Institute on Drug Abuse (NIDA). 2009. "NIDA InfoFacts: Inhalants." Available at: http://www.nida.nih.gov/Infofacts/inhalants.html. Accessed September 2, 2010.

National Institutes of Health (NIH). 2008. "Caffeine." MedlinePlus Web site. Available at: http://www.nlm.nih.gov/medlineplus/caffeine.html. Accessed August 6, 2008.

Office on National Drug Control Policy (ONDCP). 2009. "New Report Finds Highest Ever Levels of TCH in U.S. Marijuana." Available at: http://www.whitehousedrugpolicy.gov/news/press09/051409.html. Accessed September 17, 2010.

ONDCP. 2010. "Heroin Facts and Figures." Available at: http://www.whitehousedrugpolicy.gov/DrugFact/heroin/heroin_ff.html. Accessed February 23, 2010.

Ray, O., and C. Ksir. 1990. *Drugs, Society and Human Behavior*. St. Louis, Mo.: Times Mirror/Mosby College Publishing.

Substance Abuse Mental Health Services Administration (SAMHSA). 2009. "2. Illicit Drug Use." *Results from the 2007 National Survey on Drug Use and Health: National Findings.* Available at: http://www.oas.samhsa.gov/nsduh/2k8nsduh/2k8results.cfm. Accessed September 3, 2010.

United Nations Commission on Narcotic Drugs. 2008. *Making Drug Control "Fit for Purpose": Building on the UNGASS Decade.* Available at: http://www.unodc.org/documents/commissions/CND-Session51/CND-UNGASS-CRPs/ECN72008CRP17.pdf. Accessed September 2, 2010.

United Nations General Assembly. 1998. Political Declaration S-20/2. Available at: http://www.un.org/documents/ga/res/20sp/a20spr02.htm. Accessed September 2, 2010.

United Nations Office on Drugs and Crime (UNODC). 2010. "Executive Summary." *World Drug Report 2010.* Available at: http://www.akzept.org/pdf/volltexte_pdf/nr24/drogenpo_inter/world_drug_report_2010.pdf. Accessed September 3, 2010.

CHAPTER 2

Historical Perspective: The Big Three—Cannabis, Heroin, and Cocaine

The use of any addictive substance is a complex phenomenon that includes the history of the drug, the social strata of society who uses it, the kinds of situations when the substance is used, and the publicity and public opinion associated with its use. Three illicit substances tend to define the illicit drug problem over time: cannabis (marijuana and hashish), heroin, and cocaine.

CANNABIS (MARIJUANA AND HASHISH)

Cannabis (marijuana and hashish) has generated much controversy and investigation in terms of its impact on individual behavior and society. There is strong archaeological evidence of cannabis cultivation in China by 4000 B.C., and the plant has a long tradition of medicinal use in a variety of places, including India, China, and the Middle East. By A.D. 1000, the social use of the plant had spread to the Muslim world, including North Africa, and in the Middle East its use was associated with a religious cult that committed murder for political reasons. The cult was called Hashishiyya, from which the word "assassin" developed.

The chemical compounds responsible for the intoxicating and medicinal effects of cannabis are found mainly in a sticky golden resin excluded from the flowers on the female plants. There are three basic preparations of cannabis: bhang, ganja, and charas. Bhang, the least potent of the three, contains crushed leaf, seed, and stem material, while ganja is twice as potent and is prepared from the resin-producing flowering tops. Charas, also known as hashish, is the pure resin. Any of these preparations can be smoked, eaten, or mixed in drinks.

Cannabis has been used as an analgesic; a topical anesthetic for the mouth and tongue; and for the treatment of tetanus, neuralgia, dysmenorrhea (painful menstruation), convulsions, rheumatic and childbirth pain, asthma, postpartum psychosis, gonorrhea, chronic bronchitis, migraine attacks, certain kinds of epilepsy, depression, asthma, rheumatism, gastric ulcer, and drug addiction, particularly of morphine and other opiate substances.

A considerable amount of medical attention was given to cannabis from 1840 to 1900, however, that declined by 1890. Among the reasons were the variable potency of the preparations and the invention of the hypodermic syringe in the 1850s, which made opiates more effective in pain relief (hemp products are insoluble in water and cannot be easily administered by injection). Also, synthetic drugs such as aspirin, chloral hydrate, and barbiturates, which are chemically more stable, became attractive for medicinal purposes in spite of their disadvantages.

In the 1930s, marijuana received much negative attention when it was claimed that the substance would cause users to go crazy and become violent; men would rape and kill under the influence, and women would become promiscuous. Today these supposed effects receive no attention, even in the most vigorous antimarijuana arguments. The illegal status of marijuana may be attributed to four primary reasons: (1) certain special-interest organizations and labor unions were against cheap migrant workers, so attributing the use of cannabis to immigrants was a productive means of keeping them out of the United States; (2) pharmaceutical companies interested in the marketing of profitable medicines may have seen the multipurpose benefits of cheap cannabis as a threat to profitability; (3) the alcohol industry and government, with big profits and local, state, and federal tax revenues at stake, were not interested in having any competition from cannabis; and (4) cannabis appears to have served as a powerful theme for government officials and politicians to generate support for a variety of purposes, including election to public office and the funding of government initiatives ranging from education to law enforcement (Isralowitz 2002).

After years of debate and controversy, there is an abundance of information regarding the characteristics of marijuana. What is known about the substance tends to be presented in ways that support the special interests of those who advocate legal regulation of marijuana because of its alleged harmful effects or who advocate legalization because of its helpful and benign characteristics. In 2002, after a two-year study, the Canada Senate Special Committee on Illegal Drugs reported that scientific evidence indicates that cannabis is substantially less harmful than alcohol and should be addressed as a social and health issue (CFDP 2002). Essentially, the Senate Report called for the legalization, with controls, of cannabis use in Canada—a policy supported by a growing number of nations throughout the world that seem to be saying the time has come to no longer have the made in America problem be their problem. The response from officials of the U.S. Drug Enforcement Administration (DEA) and the White House Office of National Drug Control Policy has been uniform in expressing disappointment and disdain for any policy decision that is contrary to that expressed by U.S. government officials, who call for more research and information gathering on the potential harmful effects of the substance. The bill to reform Canadian marijuana laws never passed. It was reintroduced in 2004 but never got past the committee stage. The Conservative government elected in January 2006 has said it does not plan to reintroduce the bill. Additional details about this drug are provided in the "Cannabis (Marijuana/Hashish)" section of the Key Issues and Controversies chapter.

Heroin

If one substance were to be labeled the king of illegal drugs, most people would say it is heroin. Since the turn of the century when it was created, heroin has virtually defined the drug problem. "Heroin addicts are the most stigmatized of all drug users. [It] is the epitome of the illicit street drug. Its association in the public mind with street crime, in spite of strong competition from crack, is stronger than for any other drug. The stereotype of the 'junkie' is that he or she is by nature a lowlife, an outcast, a dweller in the underworld, an unsavory, untrustworthy character to be avoided at almost any cost" (Goode 1989, 226).

Heroin is chemically derived from morphine, which in turn comes from the opium poppy, which is grown primarily in Afghanistan, Pakistan, and Iran, which are collectively called "the Golden Crescent"; portions of Thailand, Laos, and Burma (also known as Myanmar), called "the Golden Triangle"; the Middle East, most notably Lebanon; and Latin American countries, including Colombia and Mexico. Opium is the product of the poppy plant (*Papaver somniferum*), an annual plant with a long-stemmed flower that is usually purple, red, pink, white, or scarlet, depending on the species. The plant grows in mountainous areas, although not at very high altitudes. Once the flower opens, the bulb is slashed or punctured with a three-pronged knife and the flowing juice, once dried by the wind, is collected. This dried substance is then boiled until it becomes a mass of raw opium called "black." Black is then refined to a morphine base, which is later transformed into heroin. Each successive step requires more sophisticated laboratory techniques, although the first steps can be made directly in the fields, where a good part of the opium is consumed, often eaten by natives in the areas where the plant is grown. The DEA document "Poppy Cultivation and Heroin Processing in Southeast Asia" provides a detailed description of the process (DEA 2001).

The word "opium" is derived from the Greek word for juice, and literary critics have suggested that the sailors who accompanied Ulysses in the Odyssey, whom Homer described in the ninth century B.C. as eating lotus, were actually consuming opium. According to this version, the country of the Lotophagi would be located in the Far East.

> The first historical reference to opium is on a wall plaque from 2000 B.C. found in Kurgia, Turkey. Opium and the opium poppy had been known to the Chinese well before the year 1000 when it was primarily used by a select, elite group. Over the years, the Chinese developed the habit of smoking tobacco and eating opium. Eventually, these two pleasures became one (that is, in the form of smoking) and opium became the substance of choice. Arab merchants trading in the Silk Route knew it as "amdak" and they introduced it to the West as a medicinal plant in the 7th and 8th centuries A.D. Opium preparations were part of the armamentarium of every self-respecting Arab doctor in a period when Arab medicine was probably the best in the world. Opium over time has been used against malaria, colitis, and pain. (Telias 1991)

By 1729, the use of opium in China was so prevalent that a law was introduced mandating that opium shop owners be strangled. Once opium for nonmedical purposes was outlawed, it was necessary for the drug to be smuggled in from India, where poppy plantations were abundant (Scott 1969). The economic stakes were high for those involved; smugglers included British adventurers and members of the East India Company. It has been noted that "the British had very little success with introducing alcohol either in India or the Far East. A certain percentage of the Asian population has enzyme systems that cause them to have side effects from the ingestion of alcohol. Thus, until recently, alcohol was not popular in [that region of the world]. The British decided to go into the opium business, and they were joined by all the other Western powers. They grew opium in India and exported it to China" (Harris 1993). When an effort was made in 1839 to suppress the smuggling of opium into China, relations among nations and peoples became strained, resulting in the Opium War of 1839, which lasted for about two years. "As victors, the British were given the island of Hong Kong, broad trading rights, and $6 million to reimburse the merchants whose opium had been destroyed" (Ksir et al. 2008). Not until 1906, through the British Parliament, was legislative action taken to stem the opium trade, but by that time problem behavior related to opium addiction was no secret, especially among those who provided the substance. At the end of World War II, there were hundreds of thousands of opiate-dependent people in China, who until recently, had disappeared from view because of strict government controls.

In 1806, a young German scientist by the name of Frederich Sertürner published a report on his isolation of the primary active ingredient in opium—an ingredient 10 times more potent than opium itself. Sertürner named it "morphium" after Morpheus, the god of dreams. Two major developments during the 19th century promoted the widespread use of morphine. First, in 1853 Dr. Alexander Wood perfected the use of the hypodermic syringe, making it possible to introduce morphine directly into the blood stream or body tissue rather than the slower process of eating opium or morphine and waiting for it to be absorbed through the gastrointestinal tract. The second factor was the use of morphine as a pain-relief agent for casualties of the American Civil War (1861–1865), the Prussian-Austrian War (1866), and the Franco-Prussian War (1870–1871) (Ksir et al. 2008).

In 1874, a chemical bonding process for morphine was discovered that produced heroin—a substance about three times as potent as morphine. Initially marketed by Bayer Laboratories of Germany in 1898 as a nonaddictive substitute for codeine, derived from opium, it took nearly a decade of research before it was found that heroin was the most addictive of the opiates, able to affect brain functioning faster than anything yet known. Despite a growing problem of opiate dependence arising from unrestrained distribution of opium derivatives within the medical system in the United States, it was the street use of the opiates and cocaine that generated public and professional concern in their habit-forming properties. After the American Civil War, a host of factors led to legislative attempts to control the spread of drug use: increased Chinese immigration on the West Coast, which was linked to smoking opium, the possession of opium pipes, and the maintenance of opium dens; the addicted Civil War soldiers; and the widespread use of patent medicines that contained alcohol and/or opiates such as opium or morphine and that could be legally purchased at a store or through mail-order firms like Sears Roebuck (Nadelmann 1993).

Although estimates varied, it was generally believed that the total number of addicts never exceeded a quarter of a million, divided evenly between medical and street dependence. Increased awareness brought about by crusades waged among law enforcement officials against the street use of opiates and cocaine aroused public anxiety about a narcotics problem of major proportions. The movement for national alcohol prohibition further sensitized the public to a need for national drug prohibitions; the culmination was the passage of the Harrison Narcotics Act of 1914 in the United States, which restricted the nonmedical use of opiates and precipitated the need for treatments to assist those who were addicted to opiates but could no longer obtain them from their physicians (McCann et al. 1994).

After World War II, anti-opium laws in many parts of Asia suppressed the availability of opium at the cost of stimulating the creation of domestic heroin industries and substantial increases in heroin use. A similar situation occurred in the United States when Congress banned opium imports in 1909. At the turn of the century,

> despite the virtual absence of any controls on availability, the proportion of Americans addicted to opiates was only two to three times greater than today...The typical addict was not a young black ghetto resident but a middle-class white Southern women or a West Coast Chinese immigrant. The violence, death, disease, and crime that we today associate with drug use barely existed, and many medical authorities regarded opiate addiction as far less destructive than alcoholism...Many opiate addicts, perhaps most, managed to lead relatively normal lives and kept their addictions secret even from close friends and relatives. (Nadelmann 1993, 45)

With a ban on opiates, new forces entered the market, namely the illegal organizations interested in making a quick profit. Those organizations succeeded in popularizing the opiates in the United States and Europe much faster than the British had succeeded in China. Until the mid-1960s, laboratory facilities to transform morphine base into heroin were available only in Europe and the United States. This meant that most of the product had to be transported to be refined, and the refining process put a great deal of money into Western hands. In the mid-1960s two apparently unrelated episodes changed the situation. Under American pressure, the Turkish government agreed to close most of the illegal fields in that country, reserving a small portion of the product for legal medicinal purposes. Also, Hong Kong–based drug entrepreneurs succeeded in establishing a series of laboratories in the field along the Mekong River. They started refining the product locally, possibly for profit from the American soldiers coming to the area and to support the war effort. It is claimed that the political turmoil in Vietnam at the time was related, at least partially, to the war for domination of the heroin market (Telias 1991, 6).

In many places, heroin has gotten cheaper, purer, and easier to find than before. For example, the price has dropped to a level that is cheap enough to smoke or snort the substance instead of injecting it, making it attractive for those who want to experiment. One reason for this is geopolitics. Since the end of the cold war, drugs have been financing some of the religious and ethnic conflicts in the world. Over time, about 1–1.5 percent of all Americans have tried heroin at least once in their lives, and among all episodes of illegal drug use, only 1 percent involve heroin. Presently, about 3.8 million U.S. residents aged 12 years or older have used heroin at least once in their lifetime; approximately 453,000 reported past year and 213,000 reported past month heroin use (Office of National Drug Control Policy 2010).

> For the past several years, the heroin market in the United States was generally divided along the Mississippi River. To the west of the Mississippi River, black tar heroin and, to a lesser extent, brown powder heroin from Mexico were the primary types available. To the east of the Mississippi, white powder heroin, primarily from Colombia, but also from Southwest and Southeast Asia, was the primary type of heroin available. While users in both markets historically have been reluctant to switch heroin types, law enforcement reporting indicates that Mexican heroin is now available in more markets east of the Mississippi than traditionally has been the case. (U.S. National Drug Intelligence Center 2006)

According to the US National Drug Intelligence Center the demand for heroin has stabilized; however, various techniques have been used by dealers to gain market share, including giving away free heroin, using brand names to establish repeat customers, and combining heroin with fentanyl, a synthetic opioid 50 times more powerful than heroin. Cheese heroin or starter heroin, a combination of black tar heroin and ground-up cold medicine (e.g., Tylenol PM) containing acetaminophen and diphenhydramine, has caused injury and death mostly among adolescents in Texas and other parts of the country since 2005. And, like elsewhere, heroin use in the United States generates considerable concern because injection equipment is often shared without proper sterilization. Viruses such as human immunodeficiency virus (HIV) and hepatitis C are prevalent among those who inject heroin.

In Europe, heroin use has long been the biggest source of Europe's drug-related crime and medical problems, including acquired immunodeficiency syndrome (AIDS) and hepatitis from shared needles. The average prevalence of problem opioid use is about 0.05 percent of the population aged 15–64 years. This translates into some 1.4 million problem opioid users in the European Union and Norway (EMCDDA 2009).

Cocaine

Sherlock Holmes "took his bottle... and hypodermic syringe and thrust the sharp point home, pressed down the tiny piston... with a sigh of satisfaction.... 'Which is it today,' he was asked, 'morphine or cocaine?'... 'It is cocaine... care to try it?' " (Doyle 1938). Poverty-stricken, Freud took cocaine powder and found that it made him cheerful, as if he had few worries, and did not result in a loss of energy. In 1884, he wrote that he used very small doses of cocaine regularly and recommended the drug as a local anesthetic, an aphrodisiac, and a means of treating depression, alcoholism, and morphine addiction. Freud used cocaine for three years, during which time he also supplied it to patients, fellow doctors, and medical students. At that time cocaine was available over the counter at pharmacies in many countries. By 1887, Freud had changed his mind on the merits of cocaine and wrote that it was much more dangerous for public health than morphine (Brain and Coward 1989).

Categorized as a stimulant, cocaine dates back more than 2,000 years to the Andes Mountains in South America. Evidence of the use of coca leaves has been found in a grave in Peru dating from about A.D. 500, and by A.D. 1000 the coca shrub was extensively cultivated in Peru. The ancient Incan civilization worshipped cocaine. Despite efforts by Spanish invaders in the 16th century to stamp out its use, the coca leaf found its way to Europe, where its effects were studied by scientists and physicians (Goode 1989). The Indians from the region (now Colombia, Peru, and Bolivia) still chew the leaves, which contain about 1 percent cocaine, to ward off fatigue and hunger, thus enabling them to work long hours without stopping.

Isolated from coca leaves in about 1860, cocaine became popular, in part, because of Mariani's Coca Wine, which consisted of quality coca leaves steeped in red wine. Angelo Mariani, a French chemist, developed and marketed the drink in 1884, and it won praise from popes, monarchs, and presidents, including Queen Victoria and U.S. presidents Ulysses S. Grant and William McKinley (Andrews and Solomon 1975, 309). Also, in 1885, the Parke-Davis Pharmaceutical Company, now part of the Pfizer pharmaceutical conglomerate, started to market cocaine as a promising "wonder" drug able to take the place of food and make the coward brave.

Mariani's cocaine-laced wine had many competitors, but none was more famous than an Atlanta pharmacist—John Pemberton—whose claim to fame was the formula for Coca-Cola. To make his concoction, Pemberton mixed sugar, caramel, caffeine, phosphoric acid, essence of coca leaves, fig juice, and, most likely, cinnamon, nutmeg, vanilla, and glycerin; later versions included ground kola nut (Hobhouse 1999, 309–10). The beverage was marketed as a refreshing and invigorating tonic and nerve stimulant in the late 1880s. In the first five years, Pemberton only sold 160 gallons of the syrup, and soon the drink was taken over by Asa Griggs Candler, a pharmacist who made history with Coca-Cola. Associated with cocaine for marketing purposes, the manufacturer of Coca-Cola removed cocaine from its formula. In 1909, the U.S. Food and Drug Administration (FDA) seized a supply of Coca-Cola syrup and made charges against the company that it was misbranded because it contained no coca, contained little if any cola, and contained caffeine, a poisonous ingredient. In 1916, the Supreme Court of the United States upheld a lower court ruling rejecting the charge of misbranding (Ksir et al. 2008).

Available in a large number of products for drinking, snorting, or injecting, all the elements needed for cocaine's illicit status were present by the first years of the 20th century.

> It had become widely used as a pleasure drug; doctors warned [against its sale and use]; it had become identified with despised or poorly regarded groups—blacks, lower-class whites, and criminals; it had not been long enough established in the culture to insure its survival; and, it had not, though used by them, become identified with the elite, thus losing what little chance it had for weathering the storm of criticism. (Ray and Ksir 1990, 129; Ashley 1975)

In 1914, the Harrison Narcotics Act was enacted to control drug addiction. Cocaine, like heroin, became less available and more expensive. During this period, in the mind of the public, cocaine became associated with show business, including the radio, music, film, and theater scenes. In Europe, during the late 1920s, cocaine had strong connections with sex, jazz, night clubs, and high-class prostitution.

The use of cocaine declined in the 1930s with the introduction of inexpensive and easily available amphetamine substances and did not increase again until the end of the 1960s, when amphetamines became harder to obtain. Three factors contributed to the increase in availability and demand: (1) law enforcement and control of amphetamines; (2) jet travel between the southern states in the United States and the Caribbean and Latin America; and (3) liberal drug culture attitudes and behavior among people (Hobhouse 1999).

During the early 1980s, there was an epidemic of cocaine abuse in the United States. Estimates indicate that in 1985, the height of the problem, there were 5.7 million active cocaine users in the United States (NLM 2010). European countries, in comparison, did not experience dramatic increases in cocaine abuse.

Crack

Until the late 1970s, the usual form of cocaine available on the street was cocaine hydrochloride, a salt form of cocaine that is usually sniffed (snorted) nasally or mixed with water and injected intravenously. Because the hydrochloride salt is quickly destroyed at high temperatures, it cannot be smoked unless it is in a freebase alkaloid form (Cornish and O'Brien 1996). The first method of creating the freebase form of cocaine is to extract alkaloidal cocaine crystals from a solution of the hydrochloride salt and buffered ammonia using ether. (The popping sound made when these crystals are heated is the origin of the term "crack.") The second method is to heat a mixture of sodium bicarbonate (baking soda) and cocaine hydrochloride until a solid—or rock—forms, which can then be heated to release vaporized cocaine (Jaffe 1990). Though the first method produces a very pure form of cocaine, the second method is easier and less dangerous. Most crack cocaine in the United States has been produced in this second manner since the mid-1980s; the resulting product is cheap and available to poor people (Cornish and O'Brien 1996, 259–60; Ray and Ksir 1990, 134–35).

According to Belenko (1993), cocaine and crack become synonymous with the war on drugs. In 1982, the U.S. government allocated $200 million for a major initiative to address the problem. Only seven years later, the government was promising $2.2 billion to finance its war. Gang violence, crack houses, addiction, and newborns exposed to drugs in utero (called "crack babies") were issues stretched to the limit by an imaginative media force. According to research on prenatal cocaine use, poverty and use of tobacco, alcohol, and other drugs during pregnancy are at least as likely as cocaine to cause developmental problems in young children ("Opposition to the Crack Campaign" 2001). Though crack is a relatively serious drug, because it is easy and cheap to manufacture and distribute and has high addiction potential, the reaction of policy makers to crack has not been in proportion to its prevalence or its real effects on overall crime rates. This is because crack emerged at a time when there was growing concern about violent crime; poor, minority, inner-city residents were linked to the drug; the media generated considerable concern and fear about its effects; and politicians used the problem for election purposes. Finally, many of the dynamics (e.g., racial prejudice, socioeconomic status, and political) associated with crack had appeared earlier with heroin (1960s), LSD (early 1970s), PCP (late 1970s), powdered cocaine (early 1980s), marijuana (1930s), and methamphetamine and ecstasy (late 1990s).

References

Andrews, G., and D. Solomon, eds. 1975. *The Coca Leaf and Cocaine Papers*. New York: Harcourt, Brace, and Jovanovich.

Ashley, R. 1975. *Cocaine: Its History, Uses and Effects*. New York: St. Martin's Press.

Belenko, S. 1993. *Crack and the Evolution of Anti-Drug Policy*. Westport, Conn.: Greenwood Press.

Brain, P., and G. Coward. 1989. "A Review of the History, Actions, and Legitimate Uses of Cocaine." *Journal of Substance Abuse* 1 (4): 431–51.

Canadian Foundation for Drug Policy. 2002. Canada: Senate Special Committee on Illegal Drugs. Available at: http://www.cfdp.ca/sen2000.htm. Accessed September 3, 2010.

Cornish, J., and C. O'Brien. 1996. "Crack Cocaine Abuse: An Epidemic with Many Public Health Consequences." *Annual Review of Public Health* 17:260–61.

Doyle, A. 1938. "The Sign of the Four." In *The Complete Sherlock Holmes*. New York: Garden City Publishing.

Drug Enforcement Agency (DEA). 2001. "Poppy Cultivation and Heroin Processing in Southeast Asia." Available at: http://www.poppies.org/news/104267739031389.shtml. Accessed September 3, 2010.

European Monitoring Centre for Drugs and Drug Addiction (EMCDDA). 2009. "Opioid Use and Drug Injection." Available at: http://www.emcdda.europa.eu/situation/opioids/3. Accessed September 3, 2010.

Goode, E. 1989. *Drugs in American Society*. New York: McGraw-Hill.

Harris, L. 1993. "Opiates: A History of Opiates and Their Use in Treatment." In *Biomedical Approaches in Illicit Drug Demand Reduction*, ed. C. Hartel, 85. Rockville, Md.: National Institute on Drug Abuse.

Hobhouse, H. 1999. *Seeds of Change*. London: Papaermac.

Isralowitz, R. 2002. *Drug Use, Policy and Management*. Westport, Conn.: Auburn House.

Jaffe, J. 1990. Drug Addiction and Drug Abuse. In *The Pharmacological Basis of Therapeutics*, ed. A. Gilman, T. Rall, A. Neis, and P. Taylor, 522–45. New York: Pergamon.

Ksir, C., C. Hart, and O. Ray. 2008. *Drugs, Society, and Human Behavior*, 12th ed. Boston, Mass.: McGraw Hill.

McCann, M., R. Rawson, J. Obert, and A. Hasson. 1994. *Treatment of Opiate Addiction with Methadone*. Rockville, Md.: U.S. Department of Health and Human Services.

Nadelmann, E. 1993. "Should We Legalize Drugs? History Answers." *American Heritage* (March): 41–48.

National Library of Medicine (NLM). 2010. *Substance Abuse in the United States: The Extent of the Problem*. Available at: http://www.ncbi.nlm.nih.gov/bookshelf/br.fcgi?book=hssamhsapep&part=A18377. Accessed September 3, 2010.

Office of National Drug Control Policy. 2010. Heroin Facts and Figures. Available at: http://www.whitehousedrugpolicy.gov/drugfact/heroin/heroin_ff.html. Accessed September 3, 2010.

"Opposition to the Crack Campaign." 2001. *American Journal of Public Health* 91 (3): 516–17. Available at: http://www.ncbi.nlm.nih.gov/pmc/articles/PMC1446614/pdf/11236456.pdf. Accessed September 3, 2010.

Ray, O., and C. Ksir. 1990. *Drugs, Society and Human Behavior*. St. Louis, Mo.: Times Mirror/Mosby College Publishing.

Scott, J. 1969. *The White Poppy: A History of Opium*. New York: Funk and Wagnalls.

Telias, D. 1991. *The World of "H."* Tel Aviv: Freund Publishing House.

U.S. National Drug Intelligence Center. 2006. National Drug Threat Assessment 2007. Available at: http://www.justice.gov/ndic/pubs21/21137/heroin.htm. Accessed February 23, 2010.

Chapter 3

Theoretical Considerations and Risk Factors

Much progress has been made over the past few decades in understanding basic factors and developmental processes associated with drug use, abuse, and dependence and how to prevent and treat drug addiction. The initiation of illicit drug use is a necessary precursor to abuse and dependence. Illicit drug use tends to develop during the adolescent years, and the behavior is often preceded by biological, psychological, social, and environmental factors that originate as early as the prenatal period. Misuse and use of illicit drugs can interfere with the normal healthy functioning of persons across the life span—extending well beyond adolescence into adulthood (NIH 2008).

> The life course developmental perspective suggests that individual and environmental factors interact to increase or reduce vulnerability to drug use, abuse and dependence. Vulnerability can occur at many points along the life course but peaks at critical life transitions ... [including] important biological transitions, such as puberty normative transitions such as moving from elementary to middle school; social transitions, such as dating; and traumatic transitions, such as the death of a parent. In addition, because vulnerability to drug abuse involves dynamic intrapersonal (e.g., temperament), interpersonal (e.g., family and peer interactions) and environmental (e.g., school environment) influences, prevention intervention ... must target individuals and social systems across the life span ... [and consider co-occurring factors including] delinquency and criminal behavior, interpersonal violence, mental health problems and HIV, other sexually transmitted infections, and reproductive health problems. (NIH 2008)

Underlying this explanation are a host of biomedical, psychological, and/or sociological considerations such as

1. the history of drug abuse patterns and the changing population of users;
2. the recognition that specific drug abuse patterns are culturally determined—that cultures (and subcultures) differ in the availability of drugs and the extent of abuse;
3. the awareness that demographic (and epidemiological) characteristics of abusers depend upon the time period, nation, and locale selected for study;
4. the need to delineate the specific drug (or drugs) of abuse, route of administration, and length of dependence;
5. the etiology of social context in which drug abuse begins;
6. the influence of major institutions (e.g., family, community, peer group, schools, and media) upon the onset and continuation of drug dependency;
7. why drug abuse is more prevalent in certain populations than others; and
8. determination of institutional supports that promote successful treatment and rehabilitation, including consideration of how persistent behavior in subcultures can be changed (Ball et al. 1995; INCB 2010, 2–6).

The following sections cover major factors that are associated with drug use, abuse, and dependence.

The Social Order

People are often referred to as deviant when they do not share the values or adhere to the social norms regarding conduct and personal attributes prescribed by society. Although the process of identifying deviance involves the use of normative definitions that may vary over time, the essential nature of deviant behavior is that it reflects a departure from the norms of a particular society.

Beginning in the mid-1930s, the principal focus of sociologists was on a systematic analysis of social and cultural sources of deviant behavior in order to discover how some social structures exert pressure on certain persons in society to engage in nonconformist rather than conformist conduct. A person's location in the social system offers differential access to societal goals. In this means/ends schema, deviant behaviors such as those related to drug use represent a person's rejection of culturally prescribed goals and available means of success, including class-dependent opportunities and accessibility to societal goals (Merton 1957, 1969). This theory has been applied to drug use and abuse, never successfully, and it has been viewed as inadequate and irrelevant when applied to the causality of drug use.

With the 1960s came growing signs of dissatisfaction with both the definition of deviance and the explanatory variables. Perhaps the most serious attempts to redefine the study of deviance came from Erving Goffman and Howard Becker, who believed social groups create deviance by making the rules whose violations constitute deviance, and by applying those rules to particular people and labeling them as outsiders. Also, during this period, studies in the drug field shifted the emphasis from asking why people use drugs to asking how they got involved in drug use and how they remain involved. This period marked a shift away from psychoanalytic theory and a medical model of addiction to a more sociological perspective (Feldman and Aldrich 1990).

Social Forces: Physical Environment, Values, and Morals

From research conducted as early as the 1920s in the United States, it has been shown that the environment where a person lives can be an influential factor in the use and abuse of drugs. An environment that is deteriorating and poverty-stricken serves as a breeding ground for problem behavior such as drug use. Living in these conditions are people from the lower end of the social hierarchy, who are often beset with a huge assortment of personal and family problems. In order to exist, norms and values different from those prescribed through explicit and implicit social policies, laws, and methods of enforcement are adopted by these people enabling them to achieve goals that are readily attainable and concrete.

Issues such as values and morals among the lower classes and the disproportionate amount of crime and drug problems found among the poor have been widely covered by sociological research and literature. However, studies show that such problem behavior is also indigenous to the middle and upper classes. Facts and statistics reveal that drug use and abuse is a problem that transverses all social classes.

Interpersonal Relations

Family

The role of the family is a major causal factor in shaping the personality and behavior of children. The family serves as a reference group on personal and normative levels.

Since *Growing Up Absurd* (Goodman 1960), it has been common to trace the long series of societal changes that have narrowed down a household to a nuclear unit, then sent mothers into the labor force, and lastly, with increasing divorce rates, further limited a child's opportunity for receiving parenting. Throughout the 19th century in America, households provided a variety of people from whom children could draw support and with whom they could identify. During that time, the family was dominant and young persons were introduced as quickly as possible to a work situation to aid the economy of the family. Knowledge, skills, and values acquisition came primarily from the family and church. With industrialization and the growth of a technological and urbanized society, family structures and functions have experienced great change (U.S. Office of Science and Technology 1973; Sanburn 2010; Trask 2010).

Family, as well as social institutions and peers, share responsibilities as a major socializing influence. Parents train their children to conform or not to conform to particular moral standards through the examples they provide by their own behavior. Investigators of families with a drug-abusing member have identified some consistent patterns related to adolescent drug use, including the role of mother and/or father to their child. Research shows that family relations; parental roles; divorce; parent and sibling alcohol and drug use; death or absence of a parent; emotional, physical, and/or sexual abuse; mental health; low aspirations; and other factors are linked to drug use (Glynn and Haenlein 1988).

Peers

Peer relations are often linked to drug use. Such behavior may be learned through association and interaction with others who are already involved with drugs. A person's relationship with peers may serve as a means of escape from other interpersonal dealings, such as family, school, or work. Interaction with peers may also be a means by which a person can receive emotional gratification, recognition, reinforcement, security, self-protection, and defense for problem behavior. Peers tend to have a consistent influence on health-risk behavior and may be better predictors of such behavior than parental influences among young adolescents.

Studies show that a high level of adolescent peer activity predicts drug use. The more young people are isolated and alienated from their parents and the more involved they are with peers, the greater the likelihood that they will experiment with drugs. Users tend to be friends of users, and the selective peer-group interaction and socialization constitutes the single-most powerful influence related to drug use among young people regardless of social class (Kandel 1980; Needle et al. 1986). Strong bonds to family and school, however, usually decrease the influence of antisocial peers.

Education

School is a major agent of status definition in society and has a critical role in the socialization process. The school labels youth as winners or losers and by so doing frequently determines the directions they take that may involve the use of drugs.

Many studies have shown a strong relationship between a negative school experience and drug use. Long-term studies have shown that school performance is strongly associated with early drop out, cigarette use, use of alcohol and illicit drugs, sexual activity, pregnancy, delinquency, suicidal thoughts, and weapons use (Isralowitz 2002).

Media

Since the 1920s when motion pictures became a major source of mass entertainment, the effects of the media have been subject to scientific inquiry and public concern. As early as 1954, a Gallup poll found that seven out of ten American adults attributed the postwar rise in problem behavior among youth at least in part to the media (Klapper 1960). Testimony before a U.S. Senate subcommittee in 1955 reported that television was serving as a preparatory school for antisocial activity. The causal connection between media and problem behavior has been the subject of more than 1,000 studies, including a Surgeon General's special report in 1972 and a National Institute of Mental Health report 10 years later (Pearl, Bouthilet, and Lazar 1982; Isralowitz 2002).

The media has an influence on the socialization process and, in turn, on drug use and related problem behavior. American children and adolescents spend an average of 3–5 hours per day with a variety of media, including television, radio, videos, video games, and the Internet. Behavior such as drug use in the media can have a lasting effect on children and youth if the themes presented are repeated often enough and if the behavior is not clearly contradicted by significant others, such as parents, peers, or teachers. Four basic types of television content present drug-related stimuli:

1. Commercials that feature positive portrayals of alcohol drinking;
2. Public service announcements that typically warn against alcohol abuse, drunk driving, and drug use;
3. Newscasts that disseminate information about problematic outcomes of drug misuse, including reports of drunk-driving accidents, drug-related deaths and arrests, and health risks; and

4. Entertainment programming, particularly dramas, movies, and comedy shows, that frequently portray characters using alcohol and experiencing positive and/or negative consequences; occasional depiction of other drugs are also presented (Atkin 1990; Strasburger and Donnerstein 2000).

Labeling and the Criminalization Process

The labeling process is a method that determines a person's fate. It tends to reinforce problem behavior rather than ameliorate it. Essentially, labeling theories are less interested in a person's problem behavior and characteristics than in the criminalization process—apprehending and punishing law violators and leaving them with a negative status.

In terms of drug use, a consistent pattern of events tends to take place, resulting in a feedback cycle involving more deviations, more penalties, and still more deviations. Hostilities and resentment are built up and culminate in official reactions that label and stigmatize the drug user, thereby justifying even greater penalties and restricting opportunities for the person to change problem behavior. Often, the drug user ultimately accepts her status and develops a career of systematic norm violations. Based on the labeling and criminalization process, therefore, the treatment of drug offenders may serve as a self-fulfilling prophecy. It forecloses noncriminal options and coerces users into a permanent state of drug use and other violations.

The roots of the labeling and criminalization process go right to the heart of a major controversy regarding the drug scene—that is, the belief that the judicial and law enforcement decision-making process underlying the drug problem is racially biased. American lawyers, clergy, and drug experts have asserted that America's criminal justice system has turned into an apartheid-like device with incarceration rising to the highest rate in the world. In many city neighborhoods, black men have nearly a one-third chance of being incarcerated at some point in their lives, and the majority without a high school diploma have spent time in prison by the time they reach their mid-thirties (Herbert 2010).

Biological and Psychological Characteristics

Biological

Research has shown that genetic factors are estimated to contribute 40 to 60 percent of a person's vulnerability to addiction, but this includes the contribution of combined genetic-environmental interactions. Drug addiction is a brain disease. Although initial drug use might be voluntary, once this addiction develops control is markedly disrupted. It has been found that genetic influences are stronger for abuse of some drugs than for others and that abusing one category of drugs, such as sedatives, stimulants, opiates, or heroin, is associated with a marked increase in the probability of abusing every other category of drugs. Heroin is the drug with the greatest influence for abuse (Tsuang et al. 1998; Volkow 2005).

The National Institute of Drug Abuse, based on research of marijuana and cocaine use by female twins, reports that genetic factors play a major role in the progression from drug use to abuse and dependence. Other studies suggest that genetic factors from drug abuse are stronger in males than females (Zikler 1999).

Another theory postulates metabolic imbalance as a possible cause of drug abuse—specifically, narcotic addiction. Whether drug users and abusers are at higher risk of suffering some metabolic imbalance is not widely known; however, there are some related factors. For example, drug-abusing patients tend to have higher rates of diabetes complications, each type of drug abuse has a unique profile of toxicity, and nutritional deficiency together with drug abuse tends to increase the risk of developing a metabolic disorder. The best that can be said about this theory is that the treatment program based on it may help some addicts.

Psychological

Psychological theories associated with drug use may be categorized into two groups—those that emphasize the mechanism of reinforcement and those that stress personality differences between people who use and are dependent on drugs and those who abstain.

Research shows that drugs have addicting reinforcement properties independent of personality factors—and this reinforcement can be positive and negative. Positive reinforcement occurs when a person receives a pleasurable sensation and, because of this, is motivated to repeat what caused it. Negative reinforcement occurs when a person does something to seek relief or to avoid pain and to feel normal (Goode 1989).

Personality pathology, defect, or inadequacy is another theoretical approach. The inadequate personality approach posits that the emotional or psychological nature of certain people leads them to drug use. Drugs are used to escape reality and avoid problems. This personality type lacks responsibility, independence, and the ability to defer pleasurable gratification for the sake of achieving long-range goals. Other personal characteristics include low self-esteem and feelings of self-derogation brought about by peer rejection, parental neglect, school failure, impaired sex-role identity, ego deficiencies, low coping abilities, and coping mechanisms that are socially devalued and/or are otherwise self-defeating (Petraitis et al. 1998). Other characteristics include being less religious, less attached to parents and family, less achievement oriented, and less cautious as well as having a higher level of sexual activity.

Conclusion

A number of theoretical approaches about drug use have been presented. Many factors, alone or in combination, influence or are associated with drug use. These include (1) societal issues of normative structure, deviance definitions, and resources allocation; (2) sociological forces of the environment, values and morals, family, school, peers, and media as well as the labeling/criminalization process; and (3) biological/psychological personality characteristics.

References

Atkin, C. 1990. "Effects of Televised Alcohol Messages on Teenage Drinking Patterns." *Journal of Adolescent Health Care* 11 (1): 10–24.

Ball, J., D. Nurco, R. Clayton, M. Lerner, T. Hagan, and G. Groves. 1995. "Etiology, Epidemiology and Natural History of Heroin Addiction: A Social Science Approach." In *Problems of Drug Dependence, 1994: Proceedings of the 56th Annual Meeting*, ed. L. Harris, 74–78, vol. 1. Rockville, Md.: The College on Problems of Drug Dependence.

Feldman, H., and M. Aldrich. 1990. "The Role of Ethnography in Substance Abuse Research and Public Policy: Historical Precedent and Future Prospects." In *The Collection and Interpretation of Data and Hidden Populations*, ed. Elizabeth Lambert. Monograph 98. Rockville, Md.: National Institute on Drug Abuse.

Glynn, T., and M. Haenlein. 1988. "Family Theory and Research on Adolescent Drug Use: A Review." *Journal of Chemical Dependency Treatment* 1 (2): 39–56.

Goodman, P. 1960. *Growing Up Absurd.* New York: Random House.

Herbert, B. 2010. "America's Black Men Continue to Face a Crisis." *Daily Advertiser.* Available at: http://www.theadvertiser.com/article/20100829/OPINION/8290327/America-s-black-men-continue-to-face-a-crisis. Accessed September 3, 2010.

Isralowitz, R. 2002. *Drug Use, Policy and Management,* 2nd ed. Westport, Conn.: Auburn House.

Kandel, D. 1980. "Drug and Drinking Behavior Among Youth." *Annual Review of Sociology* 6:235–85.

Klapper, J. 1960. *The Effects of Mass Communication*. New York: Free Press.

Merton, R. 1957. *Social Theory and Social Structure.* New York: Free Press.

Merton, R. 1969. "Social Structure and Anomie." In *Delinquency, Crime and Social Process*, ed. D. Cressey and D. Ward. New York: Harper and Row.

National Institutes of Health (NIH). 2008. "Drug Prevention Intervention Research." Available at: http://grants.nih.gov/grants/guide/pa-files/pa-08-217.html. Accessed September 3, 2010.

Needle, R., H. McCubbin, M. Wilson, R. Reineck, A. Lazar, and H. Mederer. 1986. "Interpersonal Influences in Adolescent Drug Use—The Role of Older Siblings, Parents, and Peers." *Substance Use and Misuse* 21 (7): 739–66.

Pearl, D., L. Bouthilet, and J. Lazar. 1982. *Television and Behavior: Ten Years of Scientific Progress and Implications for the Eighties.* Washington, D.C.: U.S. Government Printing Office.

Petraitis J., B. Flay, T. Miller, E. Torpy, and B. Greiner. 1998. "Illicit Substance Use Among Adolescents: A Matrix of Prospective Predictors." *Substance Use and Misuse* 33 (13): 2561–2604.

Sanburn, J. 2010. "Brief History: The American Family." *Time.* Available at: http://www.time.com/time/magazine/article/0,9171,2015780,00.html. Accessed September 4, 2010.

Strasburger, V., and F. Donnerstein. 2000. "Children, Adolescents and the Media in the 21st Century." *Adolescent Medicine* 11 (1): 51–68.

Trask, B. 2010. *Globalization and Families: Accelerated Systematic Social Change.* New York: Springer.

Tsuang, M., M. Lyons, J. Meyer, T. Doyle, S. Eisen, J. Goldberg, et al. 1998. "Co-occurrence of Abuse of Different Drugs in Men." *Achieves of General Psychiatry* 55 (11): 967–72.

U.S. Office of Science and Technology. 1973. *Youth: Transition to Adulthood. Report to the Panel on Youth of the President's Science Advisory Committee.* Chicago, Ill.: University of Chicago Press.

Volkow, N. 2005. "What Do We Know About Drug Addiction?" *American Journal of Psychiatry* 162:1401–2. Available at: http://ajp.psychiatryonline.org/cgi/content/full/162/8/1401. Accessed September 3, 2010.

Zikler, P. 1999. "Twin Studies Help Define the Role of Genes in Vulnerability to Drug Abuse." *NIDA Note* 14 (4): 1. Available at: http://archives.drugabuse.gov/NIDA_Notes/NNVol14N4/Twins.html. Accessed September 3, 2010.

Further Readings

Antonil, C. 1978. *Mama Coca*. London: Hassle Free Press.

Beal, A., J. Ausiello, and J. Perrin. 2001. "Social Influences on Health-risk Behaviors Among Minority Middle School Students." *Journal of Adolescent Health* 28 (6): 474–80.

Becker, H. 1963. *Outsiders: Studies in the Sociology of Deviance.* New York: Free Press.

Bonnie, R., and C. Whitebread. 1970. "The Forbidden Fruit and the Tree of Knowledge: An Inquiry into the Legal History of American Marijuana

Prohibition." Available at: http://www.druglibrary.org/SCHAFFER/Library/studies/vlr/vlr4.htm. Accessed July 4, 2009.

Brecher, E. 1972. *Licit and Illicit Drugs*. Boston: Little, Brown and Company.

Brecher, E., and the Editors of *Consumer Reports Magazine*. 1972. *The Consumers Union Report on Licit and Illicit Drugs, Schaffer Library of Drug Policy*. Available at: http://www.druglibrary.org/Schaffer/LIBRARY/studies/cu/cu menu.htm. Accessed March 29, 2009.

Cloward, R., and L. Ohlin. 1960. *Delinquency and Opportunity.* New York: Free Press.

CNN. 2009. "Mexican Drug Cartels in the United States." Available at: http://edition.cnn.com/interactive/2009/05/world/map.mexican.cartels/index.html. Accessed May 28, 2009.

Dole, V. 1980. "Addictive Behavior." *Scientific American* 243 (December): 138–54.

Ellickson, P., J. Tucker, and D. Klein. 2001. "High-risk Behaviors Associated with Early Smoking: Results from a 5-year Follow-up." *Journal of Adolescent Health* 28 (6): 465–73.

Falkowski, C. 2003. *Dangerous Drugs,* 2nd ed. Center City, Minn.: Hazelden.

Farrell, A., and K. White. 1998. "Peer Influences and Drug Use Among Urban Adolescents: Family Structure and Parent-Adolescent Relationship as Protective Factors." *Journal of Consulting and Clinical Psychology* 66 (2): 248–58.

Glynn, T., and M. Haenlein. 1988. "Family Theory and Research on Adolescent Drug Use: A Review." *Journal of Chemical Dependency Treatment* 1 (2): 39–56.

Goffman, E. 1963. *Stigma.* Englewood Cliffs, N.J.: Prentice Hall.

Harrison, A. 2003. "The Trial of Ed Rosenthal." Available at: http://www.alternet.org/story/14973/. Accessed September 3, 2010.

Harrison, K. 2000. "Predicting Early Adolescent Substance Use: Do Risk Factors Differ Depending on Age of Onset?" *Journal of Substance Abuse* 11 (1): 89–102.

Hawkins, J., D. Lishner, R. Catalano, and M. Howard. 1985. "Childhood Predictors of Adolescent Substance Abuse: Toward an Empirically Grounded Theory." *Journal of Children in Contemporary Society* 18 (1–2): 11–48.

International Narcotics Control Board. 2010. *Report of the International Narcotics Control Board for 2009*. New York: United Nations.

Isralowitz, R. 2004. *Drug Use: A Reference Handbook.* Santa Barbara, Calif.: ABC-CLIO.

Kandel, D. 1975. "Adolescent Marijuana Use: Role of Parents and Peers." *Science* 181:1067–70.

Kaplan, J. 1983. *The Hardest Drug: Heroin and Public Policy*. Chicago, Ill.: University of Chicago Press.

Kendler, K., and C. Prescott. 1998a. "Cannabis Use, Abuse, and Dependence in a Population-based Sample of Female Twins." *America Journal of Psychiatry* 155 (8): 1016–22.

Kendler, K., and C. Prescott. 1998b. "Cocaine Use, Abuse, and Dependence in a Population-based Sample of Female Twins." *British Journal of Psychiatry* 173:345–50.

Lindesmith, A. 1965. *The Addict and the Law*. Bloomington: Indiana University Press.

Lindesmith, A., and J. Gagnor. 1964. "Anomie and Drug Addiction." In *Anomie and Deviant Behavior: A Discussion and Critique*, ed. M. B. Clinard, 162–78. New York: Free Press.

Massing, M. 1998. *The Fix*. Berkeley: University of California Press.

Miller, P., and M. Plant. 1999. "Key Factors in Determining Whether Teens Are Likely to Drink, Smoke, Use Weapons, Have Sex or Think About Suicide Include How Well the Child Does in School and How They Spend Their Free Time." *Alcohol* 34 (6): 886–93.

Musto, D. 1973. *The American Disease: Origins of Narcotic Control*. New Haven, Conn.: Yale University Press.

National Institute on Drug Abuse. 2008. NIDA for Teens: Tobacco Addiction. Available at: http://teens.drugabuse.gov/facts/facts_nicotine1.php. Accessed September 3, 2010.

Newcomb, M., and P. Bentler. 1989. "Substance Use and Abuse Among Children and Teenagers." *American Psychologist* 44 (2): 242–48.

Schrag, C. 1973. *Crime and Justice: American Style*. Rockville, Md.: National Institute of Mental Health.

Searcy, E., A. Harrell, and E. Grotberg. 1973. *Toward Interagency Coordination: An Overview of Federal Research and Development Activities Relating to Adolescence*. Washington, D.C.: Social Research Group, George Washington University.

Shaw, C., and H. McKay. 1931. *Social Factors in Juvenile Delinquency: Report on the Causes of Crimes*. Washington, D.C.: National Commission Law Observance and Enforcement.

Short, J., and I. Nye. 1957. "Reported Behavior as a Criterion of Deviant Behavior." *Social Problems* 36:207–13.

Shur, E. 1969. *Our Criminal Society*. Englewood Cliffs, N.J.: Prentice-Hall.

Smith, G., and C. Fogg. 1975. "Teenage Drug Use: A Search for Cause and Consequences." In *Predicting Adolescent Drug Use: A Review of Issues, Methods and Correlates*, ed. D. Lettieri, 277–82. DHEW Pub. No. (ADM) 276–299. Washington, D.C.: National Institute on Drug Abuse.

Springen, K. 2001. "Unplugged America." *Newsweek,* August 20, p. 37.

Stack, P. 2002. "Medical Marijuana: A History." *Time*. Available at: http://www.time.com/time/covers/1101021104/history.html. Accessed March 29, 2009.

Substance Abuse Mental Health Services Administration (SAMHSA). 2007a. "2006 National Survey on Drug Use and Health: National Results." Available at: http://www.oas.samhsa.gov/nsduh/2k6nsduh/2k6Results.cfm#Ch2. Accessed September 10, 2010.

Substance Abuse Mental Health Services Administration (SAMHSA). 2007b. "Heroin—Changes in How It Is Used: 1995–2005." The DASIS Report.

Available at: http://www.oas.samhsa.gov/2k7/heroinTX/heroinTX.pdf. Accessed May 8, 2008.

Substance Abuse Mental Health Services Administration (SAMHSA). 2008. "Tips for Teens: The Truth about Hallucinogens." Available at: http://ncadi.samhsa.gov/govpubs/phd642/. Accessed September 3, 2010.

Taylor, N. 1949. *Flight from Reality*. New York: Duell, Sloan and Pearce.

U.S. Department of Health and Human Services. 2004. "Date Rape Drugs." Available at: http://www.womenshealth.gov/faq/date-rape-drugs.cfm. Accessed September 3, 2010.

Van den Bree, M., E. Johnson, M. Neale, and B. Pickens. 1998. "Genetic and Environmental Influences on Drug Use and Abuse/Dependence in Male and Female Twins." *Drug and Alcohol Dependence* 52 (3): 231–41.

Virmani, A., Z. Binienda, S. Ali, and F. Gaetani. 2007. "Metabolic Syndrome in Drug Abuse." *Annals of the New York Academy of Sciences* 1122 (1): 50–68.

Weisberger, B. 1993. "The Chinese Must Go." *American Heritage* (March): 24–26.

Woodward, W. 1937a. "American Medical Association Opposes the Marijuana Tax Act of 1937." Available at: http://www.pdxnorml.org/AMA_opposes_1937.html. Accessed January 13, 2009.

Woodward, W. 1937b. Legal Council, Bureau of Legal Medicine and Legislation, American Medical Association submitted a letter on July 10 to the Hon. Pat Harrison, chairman, Committee on Finance, United States Senate, Washington, DC, regarding the position of the AMA to the Marijuana Tax Act of 1937. Available at: http://www.marijuanalibrary.org/AMA_opposes_1937.html. Accessed September 3, 2010.

PART II

National and International Perspectives

CHAPTER 4

U.S. Problems, Policies, and Programs

The impact of the drug problem on people and society is examined in this chapter. Current policy, the president's National Drug Control Strategy, and perspectives on reform are examined. A critical review of major government initiatives is provided, and this chapter concludes with a list of government and nongovernment organizations and agencies that address the illicit drug problem through advocacy, information, treatment, and research.

PROBLEMS

"American society has a major drug problem on its hand" (Goode 1989, 261). This statement was made more than two decades ago, and little has changed based on observations and reports regarding patterns of drug use and addicted behavior, criminal activity, emergency hospital visits, and violence. The opinions expressed by antidrug leaders, a wide range of respected judicial and government officials, social scientists, and commentators on social order tend to agree that national drug policy and the war on drugs is a dismal failure, a monumental error, and utter futility.

Attitudes toward the War on Drugs

An analysis of 47 national surveys conducted from 1978 to 1997 on what Americans think about the war on drugs was published in the *Journal of the American Medical Association*. The conclusion over that time period was that Americans do not think the war has succeeded but they don't want to give up on the efforts. Furthermore, they believe illicit drug use is a moral rather than public health issue, and there is weak support for increased funding for drug treatment (Blendon 1998).

Milton Friedman, Nobel laureate, attacked Richard Nixon's war on drugs as immoral and counterproductive. He wrote about the violations of the civil rights of innocent people, the shameful practices of forcible entry and forfeiture of property without due process, and the low-paid police and other government officials—some high-paid ones as well—who would succumb to the temptation to pick up easy money. In 1970, 200,000 people were in prison. The major reason for this situation was the attempt to prohibit drugs. Friedman was also concerned about the destruction of the inner cities through the selling of drugs there; the harm to users who turn to crime as a result of prohibition that makes drugs expensive and highly uncertain in quality; and how the U.S. drug policy led to thousands of deaths, enormous loss of wealth, and unstable governments in countries like Colombia, Peru, and Mexico, all because we cannot enforce our laws at home among other issues (Friedman 1998).

According to "Drug Wars," a four-hour *Frontline* report aired on television by PBS in 2000, little had been accomplished over the previous three decades to stem the use and availability of illegal drugs ("Drug Wars" 2000). Walter Cronkite, anchorman of the *CBS Evening News* for nearly two decades and dubbed the most trusted man in America, noted that in addition to the war in Iraq there was a devastating war right here in the United States (Cronkite 2006). Many others agree, the U.S. drug war has wasted the lives of citizens and limited resources; it has compromised civil liberties and cost hundreds of billions of dollars—with no one held accountable for its failure.

In 1973, the Nixon administration declared that the nation had "turned the corner" on addiction and drug use; and in 1990, then drug czar William Bennett said that the United States was "on the road to victory" over drug abuse. Yet despite those assertions, Americans—just 4.5 percent of the world's population—have the highest level of cocaine and marijuana use in the world according to the World Health Organization. Drugs are now more available and cheaper than they were at the height of the drug war. Editorials from leading newspapers such as the *New York Times*, the *Washington Post*, and the *International Herald Tribune* have criticized drug policy for years and the U.S. Government Accountability Office has questioned the drug statistics used for government statements about the progress being made to address the problem.

The Pew Research Center conducted a nationwide survey on the drug war that focused on attitudes toward the press, politics, and public policy issues. The results showed that 90 percent of those surveyed said that drug abuse is a serious problem, and a quarter called it a national crisis. Nearly three quarters of Americans said the drug war is being lost (Pew Research Center 2001).

In 2005, the Rand Corporation, a nonprofit institution that helps improve policy and decision making through research and analysis, reviewed evidence for and against the effectiveness, costs, and consequences of U.S. drug policies of the previous 20 years. The bottom line was that antidrug policies in the past two decades have not been a principal influence on illegal drug use.

In a 2008 Center for Substance Abuse Research survey asking voters about the U.S. war on drugs, 76 percent said it is failing. When asked what is the single best way to deal with the problem, 28 percent of those contacted said legalizing some drugs and 25 percent said the supply-based strategy of stopping drugs at the U.S. border. Only 19 percent believed treatment and education would be most effective (CESAR 2008). The Gallup Organization conducted a poll in 2009 that shows 68 percent of Americans believe the nation's drug problem to be extremely or very serious, and most, 63 percent, believe progress to cope with the problem has stood still or lost ground (Gallup 2010).

Forty years have passed since President Richard Nixon declared a war on drugs. After four decades, the war has had three major consequences: (1) the United States now incarcerates people at a rate of nearly five times the world average; (2) criminals, including drug cartel operatives and terrorists, have been empowered in the United States and around the world; and (3) public funds, which are already limited, have been wasted supporting drug enforcement (Kristof 2009).

Numbers: What Do They Show?

The most revealing evidence about the state of America's drug policy lies with the numbers of people involved and affected. The following information has been gathered from national surveys and reports.

Drug Use in the General Population

Based on national survey information (SAMHSA 2010) it is estimated that 21.8 million Americans aged 12 years or older are current (i.e., in the past month) illicit drug users. This estimate represents 8.7 percent of the population—a rate that has remained stable since 2002.

Rates of current illicit drug use vary with age. In 2009, the rates of current illicit drug use increased from 3.6 percent at ages 12–13 to 9 percent at ages 14–15 to 16.7 percent at ages 16–17. The highest rate was among persons aged 18–20 (22.2 percent). The rate was 20.5 percent for those aged 21–25, 14.4 percent for those aged 26–29, and 0.9 percent for those aged 65 or older. Among unemployed adults aged 18 or older, 17 percent were current illicit drug users compared to 8 percent of those employed full time and 11.5 percent of those employed part time. There were 10.5 million persons or 4.2 percent of the population aged 12 or older who reported driving under the influence of illicit drugs during the past year, and the rate of 12.8 percent was highest among young adults aged 18–25.

For years, the rate of current illicit drug use has been higher for males than females—10.8 percent versus 6.6 percent, respectively. Males were more likely than females to be current marijuana users (8.6 versus 4.8 percent); and nonmedical users of psychotherapeutics (3.1 versus 2.4 percent) and cocaine (0.9 versus 0.4 percent). However, males and females had similar rates of current nonmedical use of tranquilizers (0.8 percent for both) and methamphetamine (0.2 percent for both).

Other results from the 2009 national survey show that illicit drug use varied by race and ethnicity. The highest rate of current use was for American Indians or Alaska Natives (18.3 percent) followed by persons reporting two or more races (14.3 percent), 9.6 percent for blacks, 8.8 percent for whites, and 7.9 percent for Hispanics. The estimate for Native Hawaiians or other Pacific Islanders was not reported for that year. Illicit drug use varied by educational status. The rate of current illicit drug use was lower for college graduates (6.1 percent) than for those who did not graduate high school (10.2 percent), high school graduates (8.8 percent), and those who had some college (9.6 percent). The rate of current use of illicit drugs among full-time students was 22.7 percent and it was similar to the rate among other persons in that age group (22.3 percent), which includes part-time college students, students in other grades or types of institutions, and nonstudents.

Marijuana is the most commonly used illicit drug, and the rate has been stable since 2002. In 2009, there were 16.7 million current marijuana users or about 76.6 percent of the total number of current illicit drug users; marijuana is the only drug used by 58 percent of the current illicit drug users.

An estimated 9.2 million people aged 12 or older (3.6 percent) were current users of illicit drugs other than marijuana in 2009. Most of them, 7 million or 2.8 percent of the population, used psychotherapeutic drugs nonmedically—pain relievers (5.3 million), tranquilizers (2 million), stimulants (1.3 million), and sedatives (370,000). The number and percentage of current nonmedical users of psychotherapeutic drugs in 2009 (7 million or 2.8 percent) was higher than in 2008 (6.2 million or 2.5 percent).

The number of current heroin users, about 200,000, has been stable for many years. However this may be changing because of shifting illicit drug use patterns, including the nonmedical use of opiate-based prescription drugs. In 2009, it was estimated that 399,000 persons aged 12 or older were dependent on or abused heroin.

In 2009 nearly 7.8 million persons (3.1 percent of the population) needed treatment for an illicit drug. Of these, only 1.5 million or 19.1 percent of the persons in need received treatment at a special facility. These estimates have not changed significantly over the years. The percentage of persons needing treatment for an illicit drug problem remained stable between 2002 (3.3 percent) and 2009 (3.1 percent). Among youths aged 12–17, 1.1 million (4.5 percent) needed treatment for an illicit drug in 2009; only 115,000 received such service, leaving 983,000 million youths without care. Following were the most common reasons for not receiving treatment cited in the survey:

- No health coverage or could not afford cost (40.5 percent)
- Not ready to stop using (31.6 percent)
- Might cause neighbors/community to have negative opinion (15.8 percent)
- Did not know where to go for treatment (13.5 percent)
- Might have negative effect on job (13.2 percent)
- Able to handle problem without treatment (10.4 percent)

Other reasons cited included transportation not available or inconvenient; no program available for the type of treatment needed; and no need for treatment at the present time.

Prisons and People

Men

In 1960, the U.S. inmate population, counting those locked up in long-term prisons but not counting illegal immigrants and minors, was 333,000. In 2010, about 2.3 million prisoners were held in federal, state, and local prisons or jails. Of these,

> 1.5 million meet the DSM IV medical criteria for substance abuse or addiction, and another 458,000, while not meeting the strict DSM IV criteria, had histories of substance abuse; were under the influence of alcohol or other drugs at the time of their crime; committed their offense to get money to buy drugs; were incarcerated for an alcohol or drug law violation; or shared some combination of these characteristics . . . combined these two groups constitute 85 percent of the U.S. prison population. (CASA 2010)

The United States has the highest incarceration rate in the world—it has less than 5 percent of the world's population but almost 25 percent of the world's prisoners—more than 7 million people are behind bars, on probation, or on parole. China, with four times the population of the United States, is a distant second followed by Russia (Liptak 2008). Among inmates held in prisons or jails, black men were incarcerated at 6.6 times the rate of white men—one in every 21 black men compared to one in 138 white men. In 2008, about 59 percent of those convicted and 74 percent of all drug offenders sent to prison were black (Bureau of Justice 2009).

Nearly half of state and federal prisoners meet criteria for drug dependence or abuse, and about a quarter of state and half of federal inmates were imprisoned for drug-law violations. A third of the state inmates and a quarter percent of the federal prisoners said they had committed their current offense while under the influence of drugs; more than two-thirds had used drugs regularly at some time in their lives. And, more than 10 percent of inmates in state prison were homeless in the year before admission, many with alcohol and/or illicit drug problems.

Women and Children

Mandatory drug sentencing was enacted in 1986. From 1986 to 1996, the number of women sentenced to state prison for drug crimes increased tenfold from about 2,370 to 23,700. Ten years later, in 2005, more than 1,250,000 women were in prison or jail, on parole, or on probation in the United States, including 107,518 women in federal or state prisons—7 percent of the total U.S. prison population. Drug-abuse violations among women increased nearly 30 percent from 1997 to 2006; it was the most serious offense for 65 percent of women in federal prisons and 29 percent of those in state prisons. About half of the women offenders confined in state prisons had been using alcohol, drugs, or both at the time of the offense for which they had been incarcerated and described themselves as a daily user of drugs. Nearly one in three women in prison report that they have committed an offense to obtain money to support their drug habit (DrugWarFacts 2008).

Nationally, an estimated 1.7 million children under the age of 18 have a parent in state or federal prison. Most of these children are younger than 10 years old and have an incarcerated father, but a growing number have a mother in jail (Bureau of Justice 2010). Children with incarcerated parents may be at greater risk for emotional and behavioral difficulties, poor academic performance, alcohol and drug abuse, and juvenile delinquency.

Youth: Delinquent Behavior and Violence

There is a strong relationship between drug use and adolescent problem behavior. Among 12- to 17-year-old youths who had used illicit drugs during the previous month, 17 percent had been in a serious fight at school or work, 3 percent had carried a handgun in the previous year, 37 percent had stolen or tried to steal something worth more than $50 in the previous year, and 7 percent had attacked others with the intent to harm. Also, it has been reported that youth who use illicit drugs are almost twice as likely to engage in a violent behavior as those who do not use an illicit drug—49.8 versus 26.6 percent (SAMHSA 2006, 2008).

Cost of Illicit Drugs

The Council on Foreign Relations, a nonpartisan resource for information and analysis, reports that government drug war cost numbers can be misleading because spending is spread among many agencies and because of inconsistent methods of information collection. The General Accounting Office (GAO), the nonpartisan investigative branch of Congress, has described the data to evaluate drug war progress as problematic and says there is an absolute absence of adequate, reliable data on illicit drug prices and use.

The economic cost of drug abuse to the U.S. economy each year is staggering. It has been reported that illegal drugs are a $60 billion per year industry that is patronized by at least 16 million Americans, or 7 percent of the U.S. population over age 12 (Caulkins et al. 2005). In 2000, Americans spent annually about $36 billion on cocaine, $10 billion on heroin, $5.4 billion on methamphetamine, $11 billion on marijuana, and $2.4 billion on other substances. Studies have shown that substance abuse cost the United States $510.8 billion in 1999—$119.6 billion for alcohol abuse, $167.8 billion for tobacco use, and $151.4 billion for drug abuse (Harwood 2000; SAMHSA 2009b). This figure includes the costs of health care, social services, and criminal justice systems as well as losses due to crime, impact of premature death and disability, and spending on prevention, treatment, and law enforcement. In terms of this amount, alcohol abuse is the most costly (44 percent) followed by smoking (37 percent) and illicit drug abuse (19 percent).

Federal spending on antidrug programs has grown from about $53 million in 1970 to more than $1 billion in 1981 and $19.2 billion in 2001. The White House Office of National Drug Control Policy (ONDCP) strategy for 2009 called for about $14 billion to address the drug problem. In contrast, the fiscal year 2010 amount requested by President Obama was $15.1 billion, of which $3.6 billion would go for treatment, an increase of $150.1

million over the fiscal year 2009 level. It has also been reported that the U.S. government spends about $50 billion annually in direct outlays for the drug war. This amount does not include indirect costs for the prison system, which houses a million drug offenders, and the court system. About $30 billion in state and local funds is also spent on antidrug measures.

In 1986, when federal mandatory minimum sentences were enacted, the Bureau of Prisons' budget was $700 million. In 1996, jails and prisons cost $20 billion a year; in 2001, it cost about $40 billion a year to construct and operate federal, state and local prisons. The cost to taxpayers for the federal prison system alone, which cared for 150,000 prisoners, was estimated to be $4.7 billion in 2001. This means that the annual cost per prisoner was $31,000. In comparison, a 2004 government report found that outpatient treatment, instead of incarceration, ranged from $1,433 to $7,415 per admission in 2002, depending on the use of methadone (SAMHSA 2004). A 2005 ONDCP report showed that the cost of incarcerating drug law offenders was $30.1 billion—$9.1 billion for police protection, $4.5 billion for legal adjudication, and $11 billion for state and federal correction.

A 2009 Center on Addiction and Substance Abuse (CASA) report, based on three years of research and analysis, concluded that in 2005 the federal government spent $238 billion, states spent $135.8 billion, and local governments spent $93.8 billion on dealing with all forms of drug abuse and addiction. The total annual government spending as a consequence of illicit drug use is an estimated $18.7 billion. Of this amount, $16.4 billion is federal spending—$7.8 billion for drug enforcement; 39.5 million in drug court costs; $2.6 billion for drug interdiction; $2.5 billion for prevention, treatment, research, and evaluation; and $3.8 billion in health care costs. State spending is $1.9 billion—$336 million for public safety costs for drug enforcement programs, $138 million for drug courts, and $1.5 million linked to illicit and controlled prescription drugs. About $342 million is spent on the local level for health care (CASA 2009).

Policies

The White House Office of National Drug Control Policy: Overview

In the United States, the White House ONDCP is the lead federal agency that establishes policies, priorities and goals to address the illicit drug problem. The ONDCP's efforts target the manufacturing and trafficking of illicit drugs as well as crime, violence, and health-related consequences. Established in 1988 by the Anti-Drug Abuse Act, ONDCP is a cabinet-level component of the Executive Office of the President of the United

States. The head of the ONDCP, often referred to as the U.S. drug czar, is responsible for domestic and international antidrug efforts and advising the president on key organization, management, budgeting, and personnel matters related to the war on drugs. The ONDCP, with more than 100 full-time employees, has a major role in formulating the National Drug Control Strategy that is prepared annually by law.

The National Drug Control Strategy focuses on four major policy areas: prevention, treatment, domestic law enforcement, and interdiction and international counterdrug support. The following description of priorities and programs is drawn from the 2010 ONDCP National Drug Control Budget found at http://www.ondcp.gov/publications/policy/ndcs10/index.html.

Prevention

Demand and supply reduction activities, including evidence-based prevention and early intervention programs, have resulted in fewer first-time illicit drug users, significant reductions in youth drug use, and an increased recognition of the negative health and social consequences associated with drug use. Among the federal government's prevention-related initiatives are the following:

- Safe and Drug-Free Schools and Communities (SDFSC) national programs includes a variety of drug and violence prevention activities, primarily administered through grants to local educational agencies to help support schools foster safe, secure, and drug-free learning environments for students.
- The Drug-Free Communities (DFC) program recognizes that local leaders are in the best position to understand the drug problem affecting their communities. The DFC program provides up to $125,000 per year in grant funding to local drug-free coalitions to develop plans that combat substance abuse problems. Each grantee is required to match 100 percent of its grant award with nonfederal funds or in-kind support.
- The National Youth Anti-Drug Media Campaign uses media channels, such as paid advertising, interactive media, and public information, to educate and motivate youth to develop antidrug beliefs and behaviors and to encourage adults to play a more effective role in keeping youth drug free. Funding for television, radio, newspaper, Internet, and nontraditional advertising enables the Media Campaign to address emerging drug issues among youth, such as prescription and over-the-counter drug abuse.

Treatment

Drug treatment is provided through the Departments of Health and Human Services, Justice and Veterans Affairs. Among the ONDCP treatment initiatives are the following:

- The Screening, Brief Intervention, Referral, and Treatment (SBIRT) program uses cooperative agreements to expand and enhance a state or tribal organization's continuum of care by adding screening, brief intervention, referral, and treatment services within general medical settings. In addition, by providing consistent linkages with the specialty treatment system, the SBIRT approach results in systems and policy changes that increase drug-abuse treatment access in the generalist and specialist sectors.
- The Healthcare Common Procedure Coding System (HCPCS) encourages states to adopt the use of two HCPCS codes that are available to health care providers and states for alcohol and drug screening and brief intervention. Further expanding this tool to a range of medical settings will enable clinicians to screen more patients for substance abuse disorders, prevent drug use, treat individuals, and ultimately, reduce the burden of addictive disorders on the nation, communities, and families.
- The Access to Recovery (ATR) program seeks to expand access to substance abuse treatment and recovery support services, including those that are faith-based. The ATR program allows individuals to tailor treatment services to best meet their needs, such as including services supplied by faith-based or community-based organizations or focusing on methamphetamine abuse treatment.
- Adult, juvenile, and family drug court programs support treatment providers and court systems in supplying drug-court participants with treatment services, including case management and program coordination. Funding is designed to close gaps in the treatment continuum.
- Reintegration of ex-offenders programs encourage and support juveniles and adults who are returning to the community after release from correctional confinement.
- The Indian Alcohol and Substance Abuse Program addresses the needs of American Indians and Alaska Natives for community rehabilitation and aftercare, regional treatment centers, and treatment of methamphetamine abuse.
- The Drug, Mental Health, and Problem-Solving Courts program provides alternatives to incarceration for nonviolent drug and other

offenders by using the coercive power of the court to induce abstinence and modified behavior with a combination of escalating sanctions, mandatory drug testing, treatment, and strong aftercare programs.

- Second Chance Act focuses on decreasing drug-related criminal recidivism and addresses offenders who may return to their communities to commit new crimes. Many people convicted of drug-related crimes have substance abuse problems that, if left untreated, will likely lead to relapsing to drug abuse and returning to criminal behavior. To improve offender reentry services, this initiative provides juvenile and adult offenders reentering the community with drug and alcohol testing and assessment for treatment and offers family-based substance abuse treatment programs as alternatives to incarceration for nonviolent drug offenders who are parents.
- Residential Substance Abuse Treatment ensures that state prisoners have adequate treatment services so they may become drug free and learn the skills needed to sustain themselves upon return to the community.

Domestic Law Enforcement

Efforts through the Departments of Justice, Homeland Security, and Treasury, with support from the Department of Defense's National Guard, provide law enforcement and support to state and local law enforcement agencies. ONDCP-supported initiatives include the following:

- Southwest Border Enforcement addresses the problem of narcotics smuggling in the Southwest border region and how it threatens U.S. security. This is carried out by coordinating and facilitating U.S. government counterdrug and border security initiatives involving federal, state, local, and private-sector entities.
- Department of Justice's Drug Enforcement Administration (DEA) recently added positions (including domestic special agents and intelligence analysts) to step up its efforts to prevent the flow of drugs across the Southwest border. In addition, the Organized Crime and Drug Enforcement Task Force is responsible for dismantling drug trafficking and money laundering organizations that have the most significant impact on the United States.
- The Department of Homeland Security's Immigration and Customs Enforcement (ICE) works to improve cooperative efforts with the Mexican government and reinforce intelligence operations in the

region. It has established a Border Violence Intelligence Cell to collect, analyze, and disseminate vital information to the field and the intelligence community. In addition, the Customs and Border Patrol (CBP) combats southbound firearms and currency smuggling and operates the License Plate Reader program.

- The Department of Justice's National Drug Intelligence Center provides strategic drug-related intelligence, document and computer exploitation support, and training assistance to drug control, public health, law enforcement, and intelligence communities of the United States to reduce the adverse effects of drug trafficking, drug abuse, and other drug-related criminal activity.

Interdiction and International Counterdrug Support

Through the Departments of Homeland Security, Defense, and State, efforts are made to disrupt the flow of illicit drugs into the United States and provide assistance to partner nations. This major policy area includes the following efforts:

- Assistance is provided to Mexico for counternarcotics, law enforcement, and demand-reduction programs to advance the shorter-term goal of dismantling drug trafficking and other criminal organizations and the longer-term goal of strengthening Mexico's law enforcement institutions and expanding their capacity to attack and deter crime affecting the United States. Support is provided for enhancing the country's forensics, surveillance, and data collection and analysis capabilities; secure communications network for national security agencies; and aviation assets and nonintrusive inspection equipment for land and maritime interdiction. The United States has also helped Mexico create a national network for demand reduction programs.
- Assistance is provided to Afghanistan to improve and expand its counternarcotics efforts, including its capacity to manage drug control programs, such as crop control, through public information campaigns, province-based dissuasion against planting, and poppy elimination through pre-planting initiatives and provincial eradication of planted poppy. Efforts have also been directed toward building drug control institutions through support for interdiction, public outreach, and demand reduction, including drug prevention and treatment programs.
- The DEA's international enforcement efforts are focused on disrupting or dismantling the most significant international drug and chemical

trafficking organizations and attacking the vulnerabilities of major international drug and chemical trafficking organizations. Support is provided to allow the DEA to attack drug trafficking networks and the financial infrastructures that support terrorism.
- Assistance is provided to Colombia for aviation programs that support eradication, interdiction, and humanitarian and high-value target operations. In addition, the Colombian military and police are allowed to operate in remote regions to interdict drugs.
- The Customs and Border Protection Office of Air and Marine, part of the Department of Homeland Security, provides air and marine forces to detect, interdict, and prevent acts of terrorism and the unlawful movement of people, illegal drugs, and other contraband toward or across the U.S. borders.

Overall, the fiscal year 2010 ONDCP plan reflects little change over the approach taken by the Bush administration in addressing the nation's drug problem. Former ONDCP budget analyst John Carnevale argued that

> in budget terms, and considering the lessons offered by research, one would expect marginal changes in the drug budget emphasizing treatment, prevention, and law enforcement over source-country programs and interdiction, yet the federal drug budget does not currently heed the evidence-based course of action...The requested increase (4.4 percent) for substance abuse treatment is too small to make much of a difference in reducing the demand for drugs... [however, hope remains that the new drug czar] will make the expansion of resources for treatment and prevention much more of a priority...to ensure the strategy's future success in reducing drug use and its consequences. (Curley 2009)

Ethan Nadelmann, director of the Drug Policy Alliance, told Congress, "The federal government continues to waste tens of millions of dollars each year on D.A.R.E., the National Youth Anti-Drug Media Campaign, student drug testing and other scared-based prevention programs repeatedly proven to be ineffective" (Curley 2010). In an opening statement before the 53rd United Nations Commission on Narcotic Drugs, the director of ONDCP, R. Gil Kerlikowske, made the following policy-related statements about concerns and policy. Regarding marijuana, Kerlikowske said,

> More and more people are dependent on the drug and treatment and call-in centers cite marijuana as a major reason people are presenting for help. We in the Obama Administration are opposed to legalizing marijuana or any other illicit drug. Research and experience have shown that by widening

> availability, we increase the acceptance and use of these drugs and the harmful consequences that go with them. We also believe medicine should be determined by science, not popular vote. (ONDCP 2010)

In terms of harm reduction, Kerlikowske added,

> The United States supports many specific interventions, such as medically-assisted drug treatment, syringe exchange programs as part of a comprehensive HIV/AIDS strategy leading to recovery, and the use of detoxification and treatment services tailored to the needs of those suffering from the disease of addiction. However, we do not use the phrase "harm reduction" to describe our policies because we believe it creates unnecessary confusion and is too often misused to further policies and ideologies which promote drug use. We support evaluating individual programs and policies on their own merit, not on whether they do or do not fall under any particular ideological label. (ONDCP 2010)

Harm Reduction: An Alternative Approach

A possible way of addressing the illicit drug problem is harm reduction. This approach includes policies, programs, and projects that aim to reduce the health, social, and economic harms associated with illicit drug use. According to the International Harm Reduction Association (2006) two main pillars guide harm reduction. One is a pragmatic public health approach, and the other is a human rights approach. Both share an ethos that changing human behavior must be a facilitative and cooperative process that respects a person's dignity. Harm reduction avoids moralistic, stigmatizing, and judgmental statements about substance use and users. It avoids value-laden language (such as "drug abuse" and "addict"). Harm reduction approaches also seek to identify and advocate for changes in laws, regulations, and policies that increase harm or hinder the introduction of harm reduction interventions. The Drug Policy Alliance (2009) refers to harm reduction as an evidence-based and cost-effective approach that benefits the individual, the community, and society and a public health philosophy that seeks to lessen the dangers drug abuse and drug policies cause to society. A basic tenet of harm reduction is that there never will be a drug-free society, but there are pragmatic solutions to the death, disease, crime, suffering, and other harms caused by drugs and drug policies. Recognizing that incarceration does little to reduce the harms that drugs cause to society, a harm-reduction approach favors treatment of drug addiction by health care professionals. It mandates that the emphasis on intervention should be based on the relative harmfulness of the drug to society and that factual science-based education, prevention, and treatment are important to lessen the harm associated with drug use. Harm reduction also seeks to reduce the problems caused by prohibition, such as illicit drugs that have been adulterated with poisons, sale to minors, and drug-related crime.

A significant issue related to harm reduction is needle exchange. There is "consensus among public health experts—including the World Health Organization and the American Medical Association—and [research] that the strategy works to reduce the spread of HIV"; however, federal funding of needle-exchange programs for drug addicts remains banned in spite of President Obama's campaign promise to overturn that position (Szalavitz 2009).

PROGRAMS

U.S. Government–Supported Initiatives: A Sampler of Troubles

After years of fiery rhetoric and billions of dollars spent on efforts to "stop drug use before it starts" and "heal America's drug users and disrupting the market for illegal drugs," the issue of illicit drugs did not receive even an honorable mention in President Bush's 2007 State of the Union Address on domestic priorities and international challenges. In his 2008 address he mentioned that the government is fighting illegal drugs by cutting off supplies and reducing demand through antidrug education programs. He also proposed a new initiative to help an additional 300,000 people receive treatment in the next three years while slashing funds for existing drug prevention and treatment efforts by the SAMHSA, community-based programs working with people recovering from addiction, and antidrug coalitions.

President Obama is faced with an array of challenges, yet the White House Web site (http://www.whitehouse.gov/issues/) did not reflect illicit drug issue as a key issue during his first two years. Nevertheless, many saw a positive step toward much needed change in addressing the illicit drug problem with the appointments of former Seattle police chief R. Gil Kerlikowske and Thomas McClellan, a respected advocate for treatment reform, as the Director and Deputy Director of ONDCP. On April 16, 2010, McClellan resigned his position after a few months in the position stating he was "just ill-suited to government work." McClellan's senior policy advisor also resigned.

Among the many challenges will be to assess and respond to a host of measures and programs adopted and sustained by prior administrations. The Bush administration justified drug program cuts based on its Program

Assessment Rating Tool (PART), which was developed to access and improve program performance so that the federal government can achieve better results. Some major programs labeled "not performing" by PART were targeted for elimination; others, however, continued to receive support, such as Drug Abuse Resistance Education (D.A.R.E.), the Youth Anti-Drug Media Campaign, and the DEA. Following is a brief review of those programs.

Drug Abuse Resistance Education (D.A.R.E.)

D.A.R.E. is a nonprofit organization, founded in 1983, that seeks to prevent drug use among school-age children and youth. According to D.A.R.E., it receives funding from the U.S. Department of Justice, U.S. Department of Defense, U.S. Department of State, DEA, U.S. Bureau of Justice Administration, U.S. Office of Justice and Delinquency Prevention, corporations, foundations, individuals, and other sources (D.A.R.E. 2008). The program, taught by local law-enforcement personnel, lasts for about 10 weeks. Popular and well funded, many evaluation studies have come to a similar conclusion—it does not reduce drug use and, in some cases, may increase it.

After years of debate and controversy about the D.A.R.E. program, the surgeon general in 2001 placed the program in the category of "does not work." The U.S. Government Accounting Office in January 2003 reported that based on six long-term evaluations of its elementary school curriculum no significant differences were found in illicit drug use between students who participated in D.A.R.E. and students who did not. In spite of the evidence regarding D.A.R.E.'s failure, the program continues to operate in about 80 percent of all school districts across the United States—reaching about 26 million children—and in numerous foreign countries.

The Safe and Drug Free Schools Office of the U.S. Department of Education obliges districts to select a program that meet its "Principles of Effectiveness," which most districts construe to mean that the program has to be on the department's approved list. Because results of D.A.R.E. evaluations repeatedly showed that its effectiveness in increasing knowledge and changing attitudes was neither sustained nor led to lower use of drugs, D.A.R.E. did not make the lists. Hence, many districts dropped or scaled back D.A.R.E.

In an effort to address negative results, D.A.R.E. Plus was developed: a four-session, classroom-based, peer-led parental involvement program carried out by specially trained teachers once a week focusing on influences and skills related to peers, social groups, media, and role models. D.A.R.E. Plus has demonstrated improved success in lowering alcohol, tobacco, and multidrug use and victimization among adolescent boys (Perry et al. 2003). Nevertheless, in 2007, the Association for Psychological Science placed D.A.R.E. on a list of treatments that can harm its clients.

It has been noted that

> there is uncertainty about the real costs of D.A.R.E. [that may range from $1 billion to $1.3 billion] because there is no centralized accounting of the funds, expenditures, and resources used to support the program. According to the Office of National Drug Control Policy (ONDCP), about 41 million dollars of federal support was provided to the D.A.R.E. program in a recent year. Law enforcement assistance grants are also provided by the U.S. Department of Justice that can be used to provide resources needed by local law enforcement to support the D.A.R.E. program. Officials in the U.S. Department of Education, who administer over $500 million of safe schools federal grant money annually to state education and governors offices, do not know and do not keep records of how much goes to support the D.A.R.E. program. (Shepard 2001)

In spite of its checkered history and cost concerns, U.S. presidents, including George W. Bush and Barack Obama, have declared a National D.A.R.E. Day in April for its efforts to teach children across the nation how to resist drugs and violence (see Section 3 and National D.A.R.E. Day—President of the United States of America: A Proclamation http://www.dare.com/home/tertiary/default1b34.asp).

National Youth Anti-Drug Media Campaign

The National Youth Anti-Drug Media Campaign is a U.S. government–funded initiative to reduce and prevent drug use among young people. Through the use of television, radio, and other advertising, complemented by public relations efforts including community outreach and institutional partnerships, the campaign addresses youth directly and indirectly and encourages their parents and other adults to take actions known to prevent drug use. The campaign was initiated under the Treasury-Postal Appropriations Act of 1998 with Congress-approved funding (P.L. 105–61).

In 2003, under contract from the National Institute on Drug Abuse, Westat (a private consulting group), in cooperation with the Annenberg School for Communication at the University of Pennsylvania, conducted an evaluation of this initiative's effects on youth and parent outcomes, including recall of campaign messages. The findings, released in June 2006, suggested that neither the campaign as a whole, nor the marijuana and early intervention initiatives, had a favorable effect on youth (Westat 2003). Another study of the campaign found that youth who had already begun using marijuana were not influenced to quit or reduce use. The campaign did, however, have favorable effects on parent belief and behavior outcome measures, including talking with children about drugs, doing fun activities with children, and beliefs about monitoring of children (Hornik et al. 2008).

A 2006 review by the GAO concluded that there was credible evidence that the Youth Anti-Drug Media Campaign was ineffective in reducing youth drug use during the entire campaign or during the period from 2002 to 2004 when the campaign was redirected to focus on marijuana use. Among the highlights of the GAO report are the following: (1) between 1998 and 2002, Congress appropriated more than $1.2 billion to the ONDCP for the National Youth Anti-Drug Media Campaign, (2) the campaign did not reduce youth drug use nationally, and (3) Congress should consider limiting appropriations for the campaign, beginning in the 2007 fiscal year budget, until the ONDCP provides credible evidence of a media campaign approach that effectively prevents and curtails youth drug use (GAO 2006a).

The Bush administration disregarded the Westat and GAO reports and the "not performing" evaluation status from PART. Moreover, it announced in its 2009 Office of National Drug Control Strategy a $40 million increase, to $100 million, so the campaign could address emerging drug issues among youth, such as prescription and over-the-counter drug abuse, and to maintain a focus on methamphetamine use. The program received $70 million for that year, and the ONDCP, under President Obama, has requested a similar amount for fiscal year 2010.

Drug Enforcement Administration (DEA)

The DEA is responsible for enforcing the controlled substances laws and regulations of the United States and is the lead agency responsible for developing overall federal drug enforcement strategy, programs, planning, and evaluation. Since 2001, more than $16 billion has been provided to the DEA and its Organized Crime Drug Enforcement Task Forces Program leading to the disruption or dismantlement of more than 5,000 major drug-trafficking organizations.

Does the DEA work? According to the White House Office of Management and Budget (OMB), which released its evaluation of the agency in early 2003, the answer is no. The report says that the agency spends $1.56 billion each year on drug law enforcement, but has no idea whether it has an effect on its mission. It "is unable to demonstrate progress in reducing the availability of illegal drugs in the United States... [it] lacks clear long-term strategies and goals, its managers are not held accountable for problems, and its financial controls do not comply with federal standards" (Lightblau 2003). Support for the DEA has more than doubled since 1995. Yet according to Eric Sterling, president of the Criminal Justice Policy Foundation, the DEA emperor has no clothes, and the White House report should shake up the national approach to drug enforcement and generate a major reevaluation of national antidrug efforts. Others say the OMB critique was long overdue and could start a debate about how the war on drugs is working.

Drug purity and prices are important benchmarks to gauge the impact of the federal efforts on controlling the supply of and demand for illicit drugs. In 2007, John Walters, the drug czar of the White House ONDCP, acknowledged that despite billions being spent on drug interdiction and eradication, retail cocaine prices fell 11 percent between February 2005 and October 2006 ("White House Letter" 2007).

Other Initiatives

Since 2005 more than $5 billion was spent to reduce cocaine use in the United States with limited success. One aspect of this was to consolidate the Bush administration's Andean Counter Drug Initiative, a separate category for aid to Colombia and its neighbors, with the International Narcotics and Law Enforcement (INCLE) program. The fiscal year 2010 budget request for INCLE was nearly $1.2 billion, incorporating roughly $300 million for the Andean Counterdrug Program enacted for fiscal year 2009 (Whitehall, Adams, and Glaudemans 2009). In addition to the INCLE budget, the ONDCP continues to provide Colombia, Bolivia, and Peru with hundreds of millions of dollars for drug-related efforts.

In 2007, the GAO published a report, *U.S. Assistance Has Helped Mexican Counternarcotics Efforts, but the Flow of Illicit Drugs into the United States Remains High* (Ford 2007). The reports states that "each year hundreds of tons of cocaine, heroin, marijuana, and methamphetamine flow into the United States from Mexico, while seizures in Mexico and along the U.S.-Mexico border have been relatively small in recent years." The estimated amount of cocaine arriving in Mexico for transshipment to the United States averages about 290 metric tons per year. Reported seizures average about 36 metric tons a year. Similar conditions exist for heroin, marijuana, and methamphetamine. In 2010, the ONDCP requested $432.3 million, an increase of $109.2 million over fiscal year 2009, for Mexico to use for counternarcotics, law enforcement, and demand-reduction programs to advance the shorter-term goal to dismantle drug trafficking and criminal organizations and strengthen the ability of law enforcement institutions to attack and defer crime affecting the United States.

In Afghanistan, the U.S. Congress is being asked to provide more than $288 million for fiscal year 2009. This amount is for drug control by, in part, eradicating poppy cultivation through such efforts as labor-intensive work projects, farmer education and credit support, and seed distribution. In spite of this investment, the opium harvest has reached a record level, and Afghanistan is the world's leading supplier of illicit opium, morphine, and heroin according to a Congressional Research Service Report (Blanchard 2004). The GAO (2006b) has reported that the continued prevalence of the opium poppy and drug trafficking imperils the stability of the Afghan government and threatens to turn the nation into a safe haven for drug traffickers and terrorists.

REFERENCES

Blanchard, C. 2004. *Afghanistan: Narcotics and U.S. Policy*. Available at: http://fpc.state.gov/documents/organization/39906.pdf. Accessed September 8, 2008.

Blendon, R., and J. Young. 1998. "The Public and the War on Illicit Drugs." *Journal of the American Medical Association* 279 (11): 827–32.

Bureau of Justice. 2010. *Parents in Prison and Their Minor Children*. Available at: http://www.naswdc.org/research/naswResearch/childrenParents/pptmc.pdf. Accessed September 4, 2010.

Bureau of Justice Statistics. 2009. "Prison Inmates at Midyear 2008." Available at: www.ojp.usdoj.gov/newsroom/pressreleases/.../BJS090331.htm. Accessed September 4, 2010.

Caulkins, J. P., P. Reuter, M. Y. Iguchi, and J. Chiesa. 2005. *How Goes the "War on Drugs"? An Assessment of U.S. Drug Problems and Policy*. Santa Monica, Calif.: RAND Corporation. Available at: http://www.rand.org/pubs/occasional_papers/2005/RAND_OP121.pdf. Accessed September 5, 2010.

Center on Addiction and Substance Abuse (CASA). 2009. *Shoveling Up II: The Impact of Substance Abuse on Federal, State and Local Budgets*. Available at: http://www.casacolumbia.org/absolutenm/articlefiles/380-ShovelingUpII.pdf. Accessed June 1, 2009.

Center on Addiction and Substance Abuse (CASA). 2010. "Behind Bars II: Substance Abuse and America's Prison Population." Available at: http://www.casacolumbia.org/articlefiles/575-report2010behindbars2.pdf. Accessed September 5, 2010.

Center for Substance Abuse Research (CESAR). 2008. "Three-Fourths of Likely Voters Think War on Drugs Is Failing." Available at: http://www.cesar.umd.edu/cesar/cesarfax/vol17/17-44.pdf. Accessed September 5, 2010.

Cronkite, W. 2006. "Telling the Truth About the War on Drugs." Available at: http://stopthedrugwar.org/speakeasy/2009/jul/18/walter_cronkite_drug_war. Accessed September 4, 2010.

Curley, B. 2009. "Obama's First Drug Budget Fails to Shift Priorities." May 29. Available at: http://www.jointogether.org/news/features/2009/obamas-first-drug-budget.html. Accessed June 2, 2009.

Curley, B. 2010. "Drug Czar Challenged to Justify Lopsided Spending on Drug Interdiction and Law Enforcement." Available at: http://www.jointogether.org/news/features/2010/drug-czar-challenged-to.html. Accessed September 5, 2010.

Drug Abuse Resistance Education (D.A.R.E.). 2008. "D.A.R.E. Sponsors and Supporters." Available at: http://www.dare.com/sponsors_supporters.asp. Accessed September 8, 2008.

Drug Policy Alliance. 2009. "Reducing Harm: Treatment and Beyond." Available at: http://www.drugpolicy.org/reducingharm/. Accessed June 1, 2009.

DrugWarFacts. 2008. "Race and Prison." Available at: http://www.drugwarfacts.org/cms/node/64. Accessed September 4, 2010.

"Drug Wars." 2000. *Frontline.* Public Broadcasting System (PBS). Available at: http://www.pbs.org/wgbh/pages/frontline/shows/drugs. Accessed September 4, 2010.

Ford, J. 2007. "U.S. Assistance Has Helped Mexican Counternarcotics Efforts, but the Flow of Illicit Drugs into the United States Remains High." Available at: http://www.gao.gov/new.items/d08215t.pdf. Accessed September 5, 2010.

Friedman, M. 1998. "It's Time to End the War on Drugs." *Hoover Digest* 2. Available at: http://www.hoover.org/publications/digest/3523786.html. Accessed September 1, 2008.

Gallup. 2010. "Illegal Drugs." Available at: http://www.gallup.com/poll/1657/illegal-drugs.aspx. Accessed October 1, 2010.

Goode, E. 1989. *Drugs in American Society*. New York: McGraw Hill.

Government Accounting Office (GAO). 2006a. *ONDCP Media Campaign: Contractor's National Evaluation Did Not Find That The Youth Anti-Drug Media Campaign Was Effective in Reducing Youth Drug Use.* Available at: http://www.gao.gov/products/GAO-06-818. Accessed September 5, 2010.

Government Accounting Office (GAO). 2006b. *Afghanistan Drug Control: Despite Improved Efforts, Deteriorating Security Threatens Success of U.S. Goals.* Available at: http://www.gao.gov/htext/d0778.html. Accessed September 8, 2008.

Harwood, H. 2000. *Updating Estimates of the Economic Costs of Alcohol Abuse in the United States: Estimates, Update Methods, and Data*. Washington, D.C.: National Institute on Alcohol Abuse and Alcoholism.

Hornik, R., L. Jacobsohn, R. Orwin, et al. 2008. "Effects of the National Youth Anti-Media Campaign on Youths." *American Journal of Public Health* 98 (12): 2229–36.

International Harm Reduction Association. 2006. "What is Harm Reduction? A Position Statement from the International Harm Reduction Association." Available at: http://www.ihra.net/files/2010/05/31/IHRA_HRStatement.pdf. Accessed September 5, 2010.

Kristof, N. D. 2009. "Drugs Won the War." *New York Times*, June 13. Available at: http://www.nytimes.com/2009/06/14/opinion/14kristof.html?_r=1&emc=eta1. Accessed June 18, 2009.

Lightblau, E. 2003. "The President's Budget Proposal: The Drug Agency; White House Report Stings Drug Agency on Abilities." Available at: http://www.nytimes.com/2003/02/05/us/president-s-budget-proposal-drug-agency-white-house-report-stings-drug-agency.html. Accessed September 5, 2010.

Liptak, A. 2008. "Inmate Count in US Dwarfs Other Nations." Available at: http://www.nytimes.com/2008/04/23/us/23prison.html?_r=1. Accessed September 4, 2010.

Office of National Drug Control Policy (ONDCP). 2010. Opening Statement of the Government of the United States of America Before the 53rd UN Commission on Narcotic Drugs. Available at: http://www.ondcp.gov/news/speech10/030810_UNCOmmission.pdf. Accessed March 12, 2010.

Perry, C., K. Komro, S. Veblen-Mortenson, L. Bosma, K. Farbakhsh, et al. 2003. "A Randomized Controlled Trial of the Middle and Junior High School D.A.R.E. and D.A.R.E. Plus Programs." *Archives of Pediatric and Adolescent Medicine* 157:178–84.

Pew Research Center. 2001. "Interdiction and Incarceration Still Top Remedies: 74% Say Drug War Being Lost." Available at: http://people-press.org/report/16. Accessed September 4, 2010.

Shepard, E. 2001. *The Economic Costs of DARE*. Available at: http://www.reconsider.org/issues/education/economic_costs_of_d.htm. Accessed September 5, 2010.

Substance Abuse and Mental Health Services Administration (SAMHSA). 2004. "Alcohol and Drug Services Study (ADSS) Cost Study." *The DASIS Report*. June 18. Available at: http://www.oas.samhsa.gov/2k4/costs/costs.pdf. Accessed October 8, 2008.

Substance Abuse and Mental Health Services Administration (SAMHSA). 2006. "Youth Violence and Illicit Drug Use." *The NSDUH Report* 5. Available at: http://www.oas.samhsa.gov/2k6/youthViolence/youthViolence.htm. Accessed September 1, 2008.

Substance Abuse and Mental Health Services Administration (SAMHSA). 2008. *Results from the 2007 National Survey on Drug Use and Health: National Findings*. Available at: http://www.oas.samhsa.gov/nsduh/2k7nsduh/2k7Results.cfm#7.3. Accessed September 4, 2010.

Substance Abuse and Mental Health Services Administration (SAMHSA). 2009a. *Results from the 2008 National Survey on Drug Use and Health: National Findings*. Available at: http://www.oas.samhsa.gov/nsduh/2k8nsduh/2k8Results.pdf. Accessed September 4, 2010.

Substance Abuse and Mental Health Services Administration (SAMHSA). 2009b. *Substance Abuse Prevention Dollars and Cents: A Cost-Benefit Analysis*. Available at: http://download.ncadi.samhsa.gov/prevline/pdfs/SMA07-4298.pdf. Accessed March 20, 2010.

Substance Abuse and Mental Health Services Administration (SAMHSA). 2010. *Results from the 2009 National Survey on Drug Use and Health: National Findings*. Available at: http://www.drugabusestatistics.samhsa.gov/NSDUH/2k9NSDUH/2k9Results.htm. Accessed October 1, 2010.

Szalavitz, M. 2009. "Why Obama Isn't Funding Needle-Exchange Programs." *Time*. May 16. Available at: http://www.time.com/time/nation/article/0,8599,1898073,00.html. Accessed June 18, 2009.

Westat. 2003. "Evaluation of the National Youth Anti-Media Campaign 2003. Report of Findings." Available at: http://www.drugabuse.gov/PDF/DESPR/1203report.pdf. Accessed September 5, 2010.

Whitehall, J., G. Adams, and D. Glaudemans. 2009. "FY 2010 Budget Request International Affairs." Budget Insight Web site. Available at: http://budget insight.wordpress.com/2009/05/08/fy-2010-budget-request-international-affairs-analysis. Accessed September 5, 2010.

"White House Letter: U.S. Cocaine Process Drop Despite Billons Spent on Drug War." 2007. *International Herald Tribune*. Available at: http://www.mapinc.org/newscsdp/v07/n531/a10.html. Accessed September 5, 2010.

Additional Readings

American Civil Liberties Union. 2006. "ACLU Releases Crack Cocaine Report, Anti-Drug Abuse Act of 1986 Deepened Racial Inequity in Sentencing." Available at: http://www.aclu.org/drugpolicy/gen/27194prs20061026.html. Accessed September 5, 2010.

Amnesty International. 1999. *Not Part of My Sentence: Violations of the Human Rights of Women in Custody*. Washington, D.C.: Amnesty International.

Child Welfare League of America. 2001. "Child Welfare League of America Receives National Institute of Corrections Grant to Aid Children with Parents in Prison." Available at: http://www.cwla.org/newsevents/news010919ni.htm. Accessed September 5, 2010.

Children Welfare League of America. 2005. "National Fact Sheet 2001." Available at: http://www.cwla.org/advocacy/nationalfactsheet04. Accessed September 5, 2010.

Gallup Poll. 1999. "Illegal Drugs." Available at: http://www.gallup.com/poll/1657/Illegal-Drugs.aspx. Accessed September 5, 2010.

Harrison, P., and A. Beck. 2007. *Prisoners in 2005*. Bureau of Justice Statistics, U.S. Department of Justice. Available at: http://bjs.ojp.usdoj.gov/content/pub/ascii/p05.txt. Accessed September 5, 2010.

Hutchinson, A. 2002. "Drug Legalization Doesn't Work." *Washington Post*. October 9. Available at: http://www.usembassy.it/file2002_10/alia/a2100907.htm. Accessed September 5, 2010.

Join Together Online. 2006. *Drug War Success Claims Challenged*. Available at: http://www.jointogether.org/news/headlines/inthenews/2006/drug-war-success-claim. Accessed September 5, 2010.

Office of National Drug Control Policy (ONDCP). 2003. "Drug Control Strategy." Available at: http://www.whitehousedrugpolicy.gov/publications/pdf/budget2002.pdf. Accessed September 5, 2010.

Office of National Drug Control Policy (ONDCP). 2009. "Drug Control Strategy." Available at: http://www.whitehousedrugpolicy.gov/publications/policy/09budget/index.html. Accessed September 5, 2010.

Pew Center. 2009. *One in 31: The Long Reach of American Corrections*. Available at: http://www.pewcenteronthestates.org/uploadedFiles/PSPP_1in31_report_FINAL_WEB_3-26-09.pdf. Accessed September 5, 2010.

Rydell, C., and S. Everingham. 1994. *Controlling Cocaine, Prepared for the Office of National Drug Control Policy and the United States Army*. Santa Monica, Calif.: Drug Policy Research Center, RAND Corporation.

Substance Abuse Mental Health Services Administration (SAMHSA). 2002. *National Household Survey on Drug Abuse*. Washington, D.C.: SAMHSA.

U.S. Department of Justice. 2006. *Crime in the United States*. Available at: http://www.fbi.gov/ucr/cius2006/data/table_33.html. Accessed September 5, 2010.

U.S. Department of Justice, Bureau of Justice Statistics. 1999. *Women Offenders*. Available at: http://bjs.ojp.usdoj.gov/content/pub/pdf/wo.pdf. Accessed September 5, 2010.

U.S. Department of Justice, Bureau of Justice Statistics. 2000. *Incarcerated Parents and Their Children*. Available at: http://bjs.ojp.usdoj.gov/index.cfm?ty=pbdetail&iid=981. Accessed September 5, 2010.

U.S. Department of Justice, Bureau of Justice Statistics. 2006. *Drug Use and Dependence, State and Federal Prisons, 2004*. Available at: http://bjs.ojp.usdoj.gov/content/pub/pdf/dudsfp04.pdf. Accessed September 5, 2010.

U.S. Department of Justice, Bureau of Justice Statistics. 2008. "Prison Statistics." Available at: http://bjs.ojp.usdoj.gov/content/pub/pdf/p08.pdf. Accessed September 5, 2010.

Walters, J. 2009. "Drug Legalization Isn't the Answer." *Wall Street Journal*. March 6. Available at: http://online.wsj.com/article/SB123630239109047197.html. Accessed September 5, 2010.

CHAPTER 5

International Perspectives

At United Nations–sponsored meetings held in 1998 in Vienna and New York, representatives from 130 governments agreed to a political declaration calling for a drastic reduction of the supply and demand for illicit drugs by the year 2008. Attention was also given to matters such as precursor chemicals used to manufacture illicit drugs; the manufacture, trafficking, and abuse of amphetamine-type stimulants (ATSs); cooperation among nations to improve the application of drug-control laws regarding extradition and illicit traffic by sea; the laundering of money derived from illicit drug trafficking and other serious crimes; and the elimination of illicit crops and the promotion of alternative crop development.

A decade later, the executive director of the United Nations Office on Drugs and Crime (UNODC), Antonio Maria Costa, reported that the drug-control system has contained drug problems to less than 5 percent of the adult population (aged 15–64) or 200 million people in the world; problem drug users are 25 million people or 0.6 percent of the world's adult population. Statements such as "there are drugs everywhere" or that "everybody takes drugs" are simply wrong (Figure 5.1).

In what has been referred to as "an extraordinarily candid report," Costa remarked that current policy has created significant unintended consequences, including the following:

- *Criminal black market*—A thriving criminal black market works to get prohibited substances from producers to consumers, and the financial incentives to enter this market are enormous. "There is no shortage of criminals interested in competing in a market in which hundredfold increases in price from production to retail are not uncommon."
- *Policy displacement*—Public health, which is clearly the first principle of drug control has been displaced.

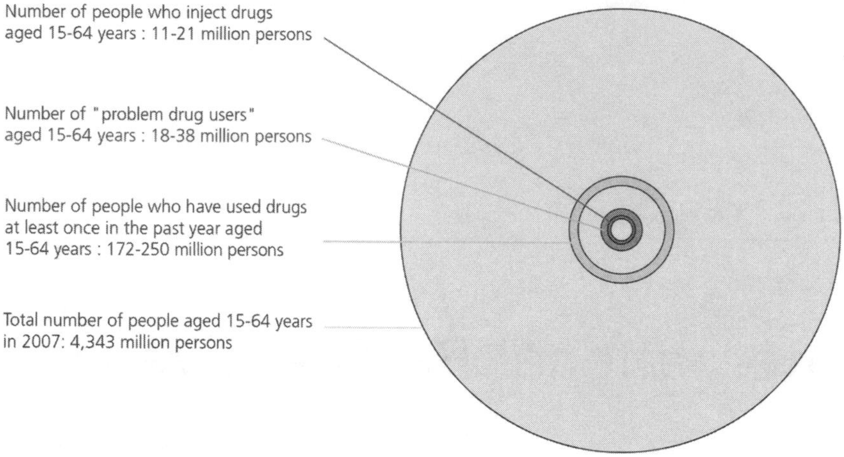

Figure 5.1 Illicit drug use at the global level.

Source: UNODC 2009c, 15.

- *Geographical displacement*—This "is often called the balloon effect because squeezing (by tighter controls) in one place produces a swelling (namely, an increase) in another place, though the net effect may be an overall reduction."
- *Substance displacement*—"If the use of one drug was controlled, by reducing either supply or demand, suppliers and users moved on to another drug with similar psychoactive effects, but less stringent controls."
- *Exclusion and marginalization*—"A system appears to have been created in which those who fall into the web of addiction find themselves excluded and marginalized from the social mainstream, tainted with a moral stigma, and often unable to find treatment even when motivated to seek it" (Costa 2008).

Another important issue raised was harm reduction. This concept has been too often "made into an unnecessarily controversial issue as if there were a contradiction between prevention and treatment on one hand and reducing the adverse health and social consequences of drug use on the other hand. This is a false dichotomy. These policies are complementary" (UNODC 2008).

Production, Trafficking, and Consumption

The 1980s and 1990s exhibited a surge of illegal drug activities. Activities such as the processing, export, production, and distribution of illicit drugs were taken over by major criminal organizations (Kazancigil and Milani 2002). In response to this situation, the UNODC was established to fight illicit drugs and international crime through a merger between the United Nations Drug Control Programme and the Centre for International Crime Prevention in 1997. The UNODC operates in all regions of the world through a network of field offices. It relies on voluntary contributions, mainly from governments, for 90 percent of its budget.

The UNODC has estimated the following worldwide prevalence rates of illicit drugs: cannabis, 4 percent; cocaine, 0.4 percent; opiates, 0.4 percent; heroin, 0.3 percent; amphetamines, 0.6 percent; and ecstasy, 0.2 percent. Other relevant factors include the following:

- After years of expansion, cultivation levels of coca in Bolivia, Colombia, and Peru, tend to be leveling off. Prices are rising. purity levels are falling, opium cultivation and production tend to be decreasing, and the problems associated with ATSs are worsening.
- Afghanistan alone accounts for more than 90 percent of global opium production.
- The absolute numbers of cannabis, cocaine, and opiates users have increased, but there tends to be little change in the number of people who use a particular drug at least once a year.
- Global annual prevalence of cannabis is unchanged. Both cannabis herb and resin (hashish) production have fallen slightly; however, high-yielding hydroponically grown cannabis is a cause of concern.
- Among ATSs, overall global production has increased slightly—amphetamine production has increased while ecstasy and methamphetamine production has declined (UNODC 2009c).

The main problem drugs for regions of the world are depicted in Figure 5.2.

The following review of illegal drug (i.e., cannabis, opium and heroin, cocaine, and amphetamine) trafficking, production, and consumption is drawn from the UNODC's annual world drug reports (UNODC 2008, 2009c), *Assessing Changes in Global Drug Problems, 1998–2007: Main Report* (RAND Corporation 2009), the *National Drug Threat Assessment 2009* (NDIC 2008), and other information sources.

Cannabis

Production and Trafficking

Cannabis is grown in about 172 countries; it dominates illicit drug markets in terms of cultivation, production, and consumption. In recent years,

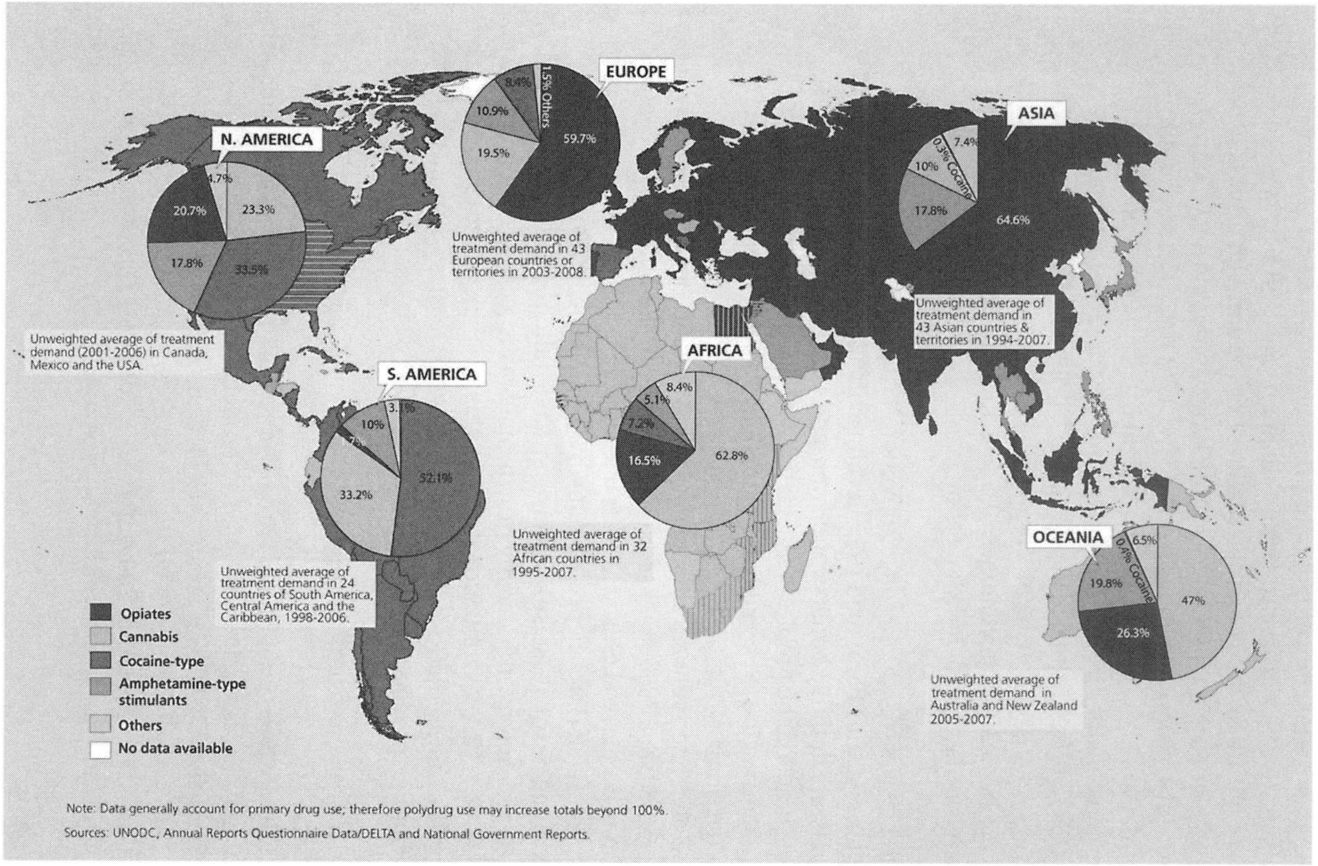

Figure 5.2 Main problem drugs as reflected in treatment provided, 2007 (or latest year available).

Note: Data generally account for primary drug use; therefore, polydrug use may increase totals beyond 100 percent.

Source: UNODC 2009c, 16.

however, cannabis has been given a low priority status among law enforcement authorities in many countries, including the Netherlands, Great Britain, Germany, Switzerland, Italy, Portugal, and Canada. Based on the declining number of seizures, it seems there may be a decline in cannabis use, at least in terms of what existed in the early 1990s to the first years of the 21st century.

In 2006, most cannabis was produced in the Americas (55 percent) and Africa (22 percent), followed by Asia and Europe. The leading production countries are Morocco, Mexico, Paraguay, Kazakhstan, Colombia, the United States, Canada, the Netherlands, and Lebanon. In North America, the largest producer is Mexico, followed by the United States and Canada. Production in Mexico is mainly concentrated in states along the Pacific Coast. Cannabis is produced throughout the United States, but it is particularly widespread in the western region (California, Washington, Oregon, and Hawaii) and the Appalachian region (Kentucky and Tennessee). Cannabis production in Canada is mostly in British Colombia and Quebec. Morocco is the largest producer of cannabis resin hashish in the world, followed by Afghanistan. Other major producers include the Commonwealth of Independent States (e.g., Russia and Ukraine), Pakistan, the Netherlands, Lebanon, Nepal, Spain, and Jamaica.

Cannabis, including the herb, resin, plants, and oil, ranks first among all illicit drugs in terms of amounts seized and the number of seizure cases—65 percent of global illicit drug seizures. In North America, it has been reported that the threat associated with marijuana trafficking and abuse is rising as a result of increasing cultivation by Mexican, Asian (based in Canada) and Cuban drug trafficking organizations (NDIC 2008). Illicit traffic in cannabis flows mainly from Mexico to the United States and, to a lesser extent, from Canada to the United States. Much of the marijuana produced in Canada, including the seedless and potent "BC bud," is intended for local consumption. Domestic cultivation, especially using indoor hydroponics, including those in private homes, exists in many areas.

In Kentucky, it has been reported that the annual marijuana crop grown there generates billions of dollars from markets in the Northeast where people are willing to pay high street prices. According to Sgt. Ronnie Ray, a marijuana suppression officer with the Kentucky State Police, "It's kind of like the old moonshine days with neighbors making a living at it," Ray adds, "Everybody seems to know somebody who grows it, sells it, smokes it... It's the dirty little secret of Kentucky." In addition, thousands of pot plants, each worth about $1,000 in retail produce, are seized each year in the Daniel Boone National Forest. Also, indoor planters with hydroponics and growing lamps are used to produce a crop every 89 days in basements, silos, closets and even underground bunkers, replete with booby traps and remote video monitoring (Clines 2001).

Consumption

Cannabis is the most widely used illicit drug in the world (Figure 5.3). It is estimated that between 142 and 190 million persons, or about 4 percent of the global population aged 15 years and older, used cannabis at least once in 2007 (UNODC 2009c).

Over the past few years, it appears that cannabis use is stabilizing or falling slightly in the industrialized countries of North America, west and central Europe, and the Oceania region. In many developing countries of Africa, South America, and Asia, however, cannabis use seems to be on the rise.

In the United States, marijuana was used at least once a month during 2009 by 16.7 million people; 76.6 percent of current (i.e., within the past month) illicit drug users and was the only drug used by 58 percent of them.

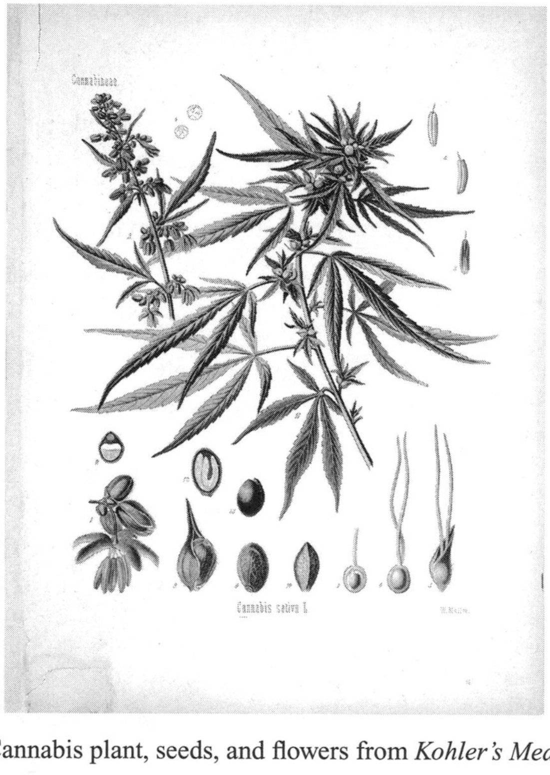

Figure 5.3 Cannabis plant, seeds, and flowers from *Kohler's Medicinal Plants.*

Source: Image provided by Missouri Botanical Garden Library, www.mobot.org / www.botanicus.org. Missouri Botanical Garden.

Among persons aged 12 or older, the overall rate of current marijuana use in 2009 (8.7 percent) was higher than the rate in 2008 (6.1 percent). Overall, cannabis use declined in North America since 2000. Males were more likely than females to be current marijuana users—8.6 percent versus 4.8 percent (SAMHSA 2010). Cannabis use has declined significantly among high school students in North America since 2002 (UNODC 2009c).

Opium and Heroin

Production and Trafficking

In the 1990s, Afghanistan became the world's leading opium producer with about 80 percent of the global illicit opium production (5,674 metric tons) by 1999 (Figure 5.4). Following the imposed ban by the Taliban in July 2000, Afghanistan opium poppy cultivation was down by 91 percent, and opium production dropped by 94 percent in 2001 (185 metric tons) compared to the 2000 levels (3,276 metric tons). With production curtailed

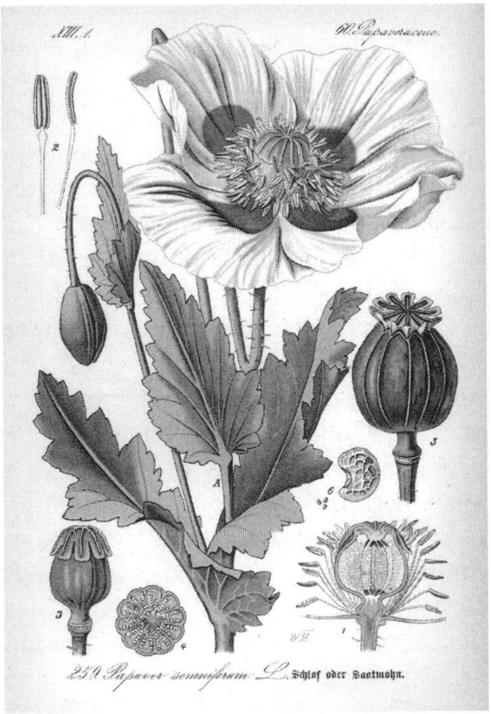

Figure 5.4 Opium poppy.

Source: From Otto Wilhelm Thome, *Flora von Deutschland, Österreich und der Schweiz* (Gera, Germany, 1885).

in 2001, an opiate shortage was expected on the West European market. Among the projected consequences were price increases, including a rise in crime by addicts to pay the higher prices; a reduction in the purity of heroin sold in the street and the resulting health implications; a shift to legal opiate substitutes, such as methadone or buprenorphine, or to other illegal substances available on the market, such as cocaine and ATSs; and an increase in the demand for treatment. Many of these conditions might have happened if it had not been for the events of 9/11 and the subsequent military campaign. Instead, consumer prices fell because suppliers panicked and sold their opiate stocks, and there was an ample supply for transport to Western Europe. After this period, despite recognition of the connection between the drug-trade revenues and terrorist activity, and a military conflict involving Western forces from the United States, Britain, and other countries, the fortunes of Afghanistan grew.

In 2008, Afghanistan alone accounted for more than 90 percent of global production, at an estimated 7,700 metric tons. Every year, the equivalent of some 3,500 tons of opium flows from Afghanistan to the rest of the world through its neighboring countries: 40 percent through the Islamic Republic of Iran, 30 percent through Pakistan, and the rest through Central Asia (Tajikistan, Uzbekistan, and Turkmenistan; UNODC 2009a). The potential gross export value of Afghanistan's opiates was $2.8 billion in 2009—the equivalent of about a quarter of the country's gross domestic product (GDP). This amount, however, reflects a decline from $3.4 billion in 2008, as a result of less cultivation, lower production, lower prices, and relatively higher GDP (UNODC 2009b). Other opium producers are Myanmar and Mexico (the principal supplier for the Western Hemisphere), followed by Pakistan, Colombia, and the Lao People's Democratic Republic (see Figure 5.5).

The history of heroin trafficking in the United States during the past 25 years is a prime example of how flexible heroin sources, moving from one region to another, can address market demand. In 1972, for example, the French Connection that had been supplying Turkish heroin to the U.S. market was disbanded and Turkey enforced a ban on opium production. In response, Mexican heroin was brought in to fill the gap. The Mexican government soon initiated a process of eradication that led to the need to find another source—Southeast Asian heroin. With a decline of Mexican and Southeast Asian heroin, the result of a drought combined with the development of the cocaine epidemic, there was a decreased level of heroin abuse in the United States.

For the next 15 years, from 1979 to 1993, heroin use levels remained stable at a relatively low level. During that time heroin from Southeast Asia, Pakistan, and then Afghanistan dominated the U.S. market. In the early 1990s opium poppy cultivation started to develop in Colombia. This,

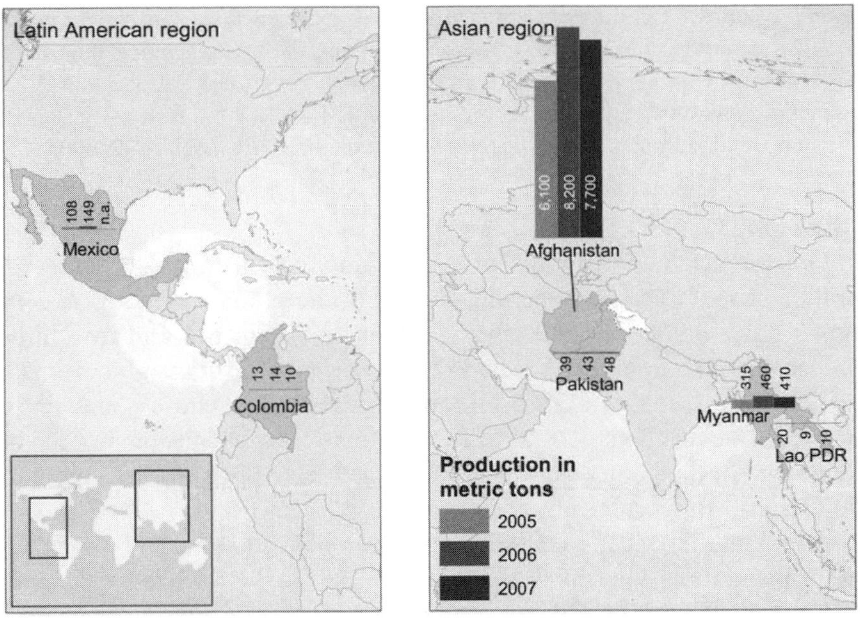

Figure 5.5 Places where opium poppy production is prevalent.

Source: UNODC 2009c, 39.

along with a number of heroin-trafficking problems in Southeast Asia provided the opportunity for Colombian heroin to make its entry into the United States fueling a revived heroin demand. In 1994, Colombia produced 205 metric tons of opium, an amount that has dropped significantly to 14 metric tons in 2007. In its place, Mexico has become the principal producer and supplier of opium to the United States and other countries in the Western Hemisphere (UNODCCP 2002; UNODC 2008).

Thomas Schweich (2008), who served the Bush administration as the ambassador for counternarcotics and justice reform in Afghanistan, provides a revealing expose of conditions in Afghanistan. The following excerpt is drawn from his article published in the *New York Times Magazine*:

> I took to heart Karzai's (Afghan President) strong statements against the Afghan drug trade. That was my first mistake... Over the next two years I would discover how deeply the Afghan government was involved in protecting the opium trade—by shielding it from American-designed policies... The trouble is that the fighting is unlikely to end as long as the Taliban can finance themselves through drugs—and as long as the Kabul government is dependent on opium to sustain its own hold on power.... [T]he Afghans congratulated themselves on their tremendous success in fighting drugs even as everyone knew the problem was worse than ever... Less than 1 percent of

> the opium produced in Afghanistan was being seized there. There was no coherent strategy to resolve these issues among the U.S. agencies and the Afghan government... despite some successes, poppy cultivation over all would grow by about 17 percent in 2007. Opium cultivation in Afghanistan is no longer associated with poverty—quite the opposite. (Schweich 2008)

Consumption

Opiates are the main problem drug throughout the world. About 16.5 million people use opium, heroin, and morphine annually. The world consumes some 3,700 tons of opium per year (one-third raw and two-thirds processed into heroin) and seizes 1,000 tons. The value of the global opiate market is estimated at US$65 billion per year. Those who use and abuse opiates make up about two-thirds to three quarters of the people in need of treatment. In the United States more people are admitted for treatment of opiates than for cocaine abuse.

The annual prevalence rate of users has remained stable at 0.4 percent of the population since the late 1990s. Over half of the world's opiate users live in Asia (9.3 million), mainly in the areas of Afghanistan and Myanmar. About 4 million, or 22 percent, of users are in Europe, mainly the central and eastern subregions (e.g., the Russian Federation and the Ukraine), where about 1 percent of the population aged 15–64 years have used opiates at least once in the previous year. The major opiate markets in Western Europe are the United Kingdom, Italy, France, Germany, and Spain.

In North, Central, and South America and the Caribbean, it is estimated that there are 2.2 million opiate users (0.4 percent of the population). Worldwide, this is equivalent to 13 percent of all opiate users. The largest opiate market in this region is the United States, with approximately 1.2 million heroin users, or 0.6 percent of the population; about 200,000 are current heroin users. These numbers tend to be stable from year to year (SAMHSA 2009, 2010; UNODC 2009c). In the United States, males more than females, and blacks more than whites or Hispanics are likely to report lifetime use of heroin. Lifetime use also is higher among unemployed persons than among the employed. Heroin use is generally concentrated in the Northeast where the drug is most available.

Throughout the United States, heroin has been used in different ways. For example, injecting remains the most common route of administration in most cities; however, intranasal use has been popular in some locations. "Monkey water" and "shebanging" are terms associated with heroin use where the drug is dissolved in water and then either sprayed up the nose using a squeeze bottle or squirted up the nose using a syringe. Because of the high purity, snorting is often the common starting route of administration among new and younger users, but progression to injection is widely reported because it increases the effect from a given amount of heroin. There are reports of younger adults burning heroin in aluminum foil and inhaling the fumes, a practice called "chasin' the dragon," or they snort the powder form. These alternative methods of using heroin are often seen in the sex industry business and topless bars. Smoking heroin remains relatively rare; it accounts for only 1–3 percent of heroin hospital emergency department admissions in most eastern and central parts of the United States (NDIC 2008).

Cocaine

Production and Trafficking

Coca is a product of Colombia, Peru, and Bolivia, and the coca leaf is the source for cocaine hydrochloride and crack (Figure 5.6). In terms of

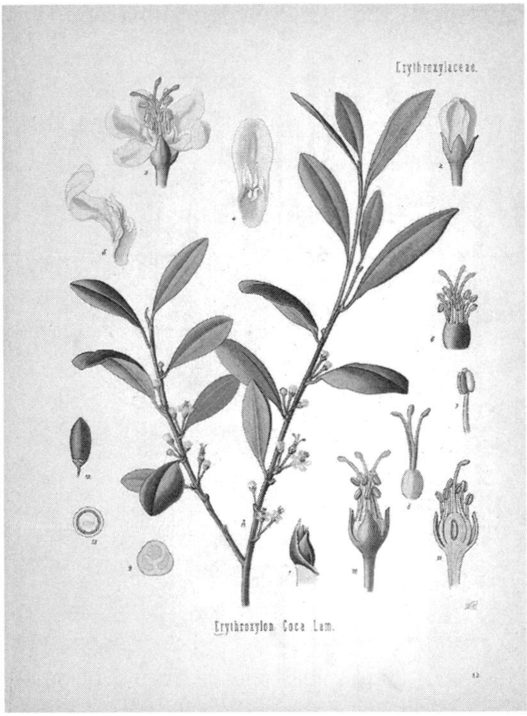

Figure 5.6 Coca plant, seeds, and flowers from *Kohler's Medicinal Plants*.

Source: Image provided by Missouri Botanical Garden Library, www.mobot.org / www.botanicus.org. Missouri Botanical Garden.

cocaine production, Colombia produces about 51 percent, Peru 36 percent, and Bolivia 13 percent; the entire manufacturing cycle is, for the most part, confined to these countries. An estimated 1 million people in these countries, including farmers and laborers, grow coca leaves and process and export cocaine products. At the growing and harvesting stages, those involved are simple farmers and rural laborers who are out to earn an income from a crop long consumed without great danger. For the most part, poor people involved with coca production know they are breaking the law, but that is unfortunately common in societies with large informal sectors.

The income from the cocaine industry grew in the late 1970s and early 1980s. Such a rise was associated with the deep economic troubles of Bolivia and Peru resulting from government deficits and rampant inflation (Figure 5.7). A vicious cycle was created for these two countries when the price for coca leaf soared while the legal economy was in a state of decline. To temporarily hide conditions, the Bolivian and Peruvian governments created massive overemployment in the government and in loss-making state-owned enterprises. With the major populations centers no longer able to absorb migrants from the overcrowded and resource-poor highlands,

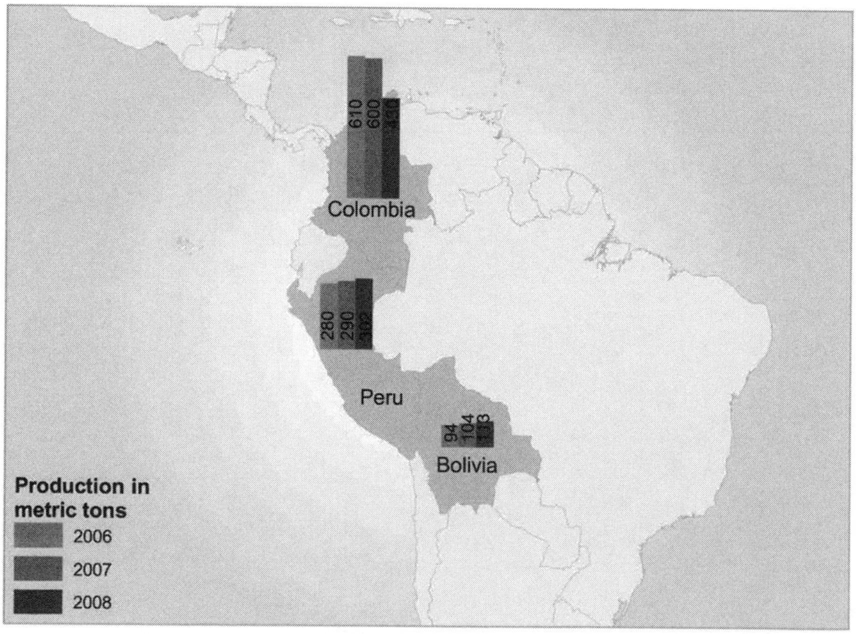

Figure 5.7 Potential cocaine production.

Source: UNODC 2009c, 69.

poor people from the highlands had little choice but to move to the coca-growing regions to grow coca (USIA 1992).

Mexico is the main transit country for cocaine shipment to North America. The main entry point continues to be the common borders of Mexico with southern Texas and southern California. Authorities in the United States estimate that around 90 percent of the cocaine that entered the country in 2006 transited the Mexico–Central America corridor and came from Mexican drug transit organizations that dominate the distribution of wholesale quantities of cocaine in the United States (see Figure 5.8). About 81 percent of all the cocaine seized in the world is in the Americas—45 percent in South America, where most cocaine is manufactured. North America, the world's largest cocaine market, accounted for 24 percent and Central America and the Caribbean, 11 percent. The only large market outside the Americas is Europe. There, 17 percent of global cocaine seizures were made. Overall, global cocaine seizures have increased, possibly because of improved law enforcement services and intelligence information. In the United States, cocaine smuggling and availability tend to be on the decline, and shortages are occurring in many U.S. drug markets (NDIC 2008).

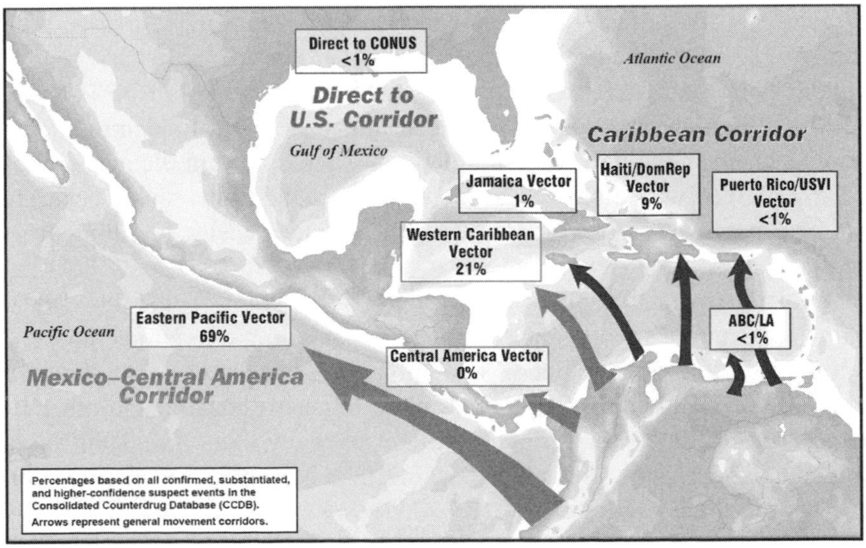

Figure 5.8 National Drug Intelligence Center vectors in the transit zone. Consolidated Counterdrug Database–documented cocaine flow departing South America, January to December 2007.

Source: National Drug Intelligence Center, National Drug Threat Assessment 2009.

The need to bring cocaine to its principal market, the United States, has generated a considerable amount of ingenious illegal import activity over time. For example, one courier had a half of pound of cocaine surgically implanted under the skin of each of his thighs. The cocaine was divided into four packages of one square inch each and containing one quarter pound of cocaine each. Cocaine has been carried across the border into Arizona on the backs of mules or horses or on foot and has been containerized and shipped out of Ecuador with such products as shrimp, cacao, and bananas. Tons of cocaine have been shipped from Venezuela to Miami, Florida, inside concrete fencing posts, in false-bottomed metal boxes labeled as toilet seats and bathroom sinks, in counterfeit bottles of Pony Malta de Bavaria (a nonalcoholic malt drink from Colombia), in 55-gallon drums of guava pulp (with the cocaine in plastic packets inside the fruit), in cardboard boxes packed with canned fruit stuffed with cocaine, in anchovy cans shipped from Argentina, in stuffed teddy bears, in Peruvian handicrafts, and in cans marked as asparagus. Panamanian cocaine smugglers have developed a technology that combines cocaine with vinyl to produce a material that has been used in making luggage and sneakers. The cocaine is separated from the vinyl after reaching its destination. Cocaine has been smuggled in suitcases hidden behind interior panels of airplanes, hidden in a secret tank in the fuel tank of a cabin cruiser, and packed in 1-kilogram lots and placed inside a plastic pipe that was bolted to the bottom of a banana boat docked in the Bridgeport, Connecticut, harbor. It has been sewn into the interior roof of a family station wagon and transported during a family vacation, hidden in a false compartment in the floor of a mobile home, and placed in the gas tank of a car equipped with a baffle that made the left side of the tank a separate compartment. A ton of cocaine was found hidden inside a shipment of frozen sharks.

With the disintegration of the former Soviet Union in the late 1980s came opportunities to expand Russian-speaking drug operations throughout the world. In one incidence, Columbia drug traffickers considered the purchase of a Russian made submarine to transport cocaine and other illegal drugs. Officials in the United States estimate that "drug subs" now transport about one-third of all cocaine that moves by sea from South America to the United States (CNN 2009).

Consumption

Worldwide, approximately 16 million people, or 0.4 percent of the global population aged 15–64, use cocaine; 6.8 million people or 44 percent from North America followed by 3.8 million people or 24 percent from

Western and Central Europe and 2.5 million people or 16 percent from South America, including Central America and the Caribbean. Cocaine is the second most common problem drug in terms of treatment demand. On a global level, however, cocaine use has stabilized as a result of declining use in the United States and Canada. Over the past 10 years, cocaine use has increased in Europe.

Cocaine Abuse

Over time, patterns of lifetime, past year, and past month cocaine use in the United States tend to be more common among males than females. When broken down by age, however, gender differences are not always found. Males account for the most deaths, emergency department visits, and cocaine treatment admissions. Whites tend to have a higher lifetime use of cocaine than blacks and Hispanics, but past-month use tends to be higher among blacks and Hispanics than whites. In the total population, past-year and past-month cocaine use is more likely to occur among those with less than a high school education than among those who had attended or graduated from college. Unemployed adults use cocaine at higher rates than employed adults. There are an estimated 1.6 million current cocaine users aged 12 or older (SAMHSA 2010). Prevalence data from 2008 shows there were an estimated 36.7 million (14.7 percent) cocaine and 8.5 million (3.4 percent) crack lifetime users; 5.2 million (2.1 percent) cocaine and 1.1 million (0.4 percent) crack past-year users; and 1.8 million (0.7 percent) cocaine and 359,000 (0.1 percent) crack past-month users (SAMHSA 2009). From national survey information, only 50 percent of persons aged 12 to 17 perceive great risk in using cocaine once a month. Among adolescents, a decrease in perceived risk "suggests that adolescents are becoming less wary of trying cocaine, which may sustain demand for the drug in the near term; and despite declines in cocaine availability and abuse, demand for the drug will likely remain high in the near term" (NDIC 2008, 8).

Throughout the United States the following routes of cocaine and crack use have been reported. Smoking, typically crack, is the dominant route of administration reported by those admitted for cocaine treatment. Needle-exchange workers in major cities have seen some injecting drug users dissolve crack cocaine in vinegar or lemon juice to be used in combination with heroin (called "speedballing"). Drug paraphernalia laws imposed to eliminate the sale of crack pipes have caused crack (rock) users to improvise using cans or bottles to smoke the drug; smokers have even used a car antenna and a piece of scouring pad as a screen to smoke rock. Crack/marijuana combinations are also reported in some areas, and a "bazooka" is crack and tobacco in a joint. Some users even dip crack in formaldehyde to produce a more intense high (NIDA 1996, 2001).

AMPHETAMINE-TYPE STIMULANTS

Production and Trafficking

The ATS markets are made up of two groups of substances: the amphetamines group (amphetamine, methamphetamine, and nonspecified amphetamine, for example, fenetylline, methylphenidate, phenmetrazine, methcathinone, amfepramone, pemoline, phentermine) and the ecstasy group (MDMA, MDA, and MDE/MDEA). Most (about 80 percent) of all ATSs manufactured are from the amphetamine group. (*Note:* methamphetamine is methylated, meaning that it is water soluble, and therefore more quickly absorbed by the human body, and can be injected. Methamphetamine breaks down into amphetamine once it is ingested.)

It is estimated that the worldwide manufacture of ATSs is between 302 to 777 metric tons (see Table 5.1). The production of ATSs is region specific, related to both market demand and chemical availability. Methamphetamine is manufactured throughout East and Southeast Asia, North America, and Oceania, where its precursor chemicals are more readily available and demand is high. A precursor is a chemical that, when

Table 5.1 UNODC Range Estimates of Illicit ATS Manufacture, by Drug Group (mt)

	Amphetamines-group (methamphetamine, amphetamine)		Ecstasy-group (MDMA, MDA, and MDE/MDEA)	
	Low Estimate	**High Estimate**	**Low Estimate**	**High Estimate**
Annual Consumers	15,820,000	50,570,000	11,580,000	23,510,000
Average Consumption (grams/ annually)	11.8	11.8	5.45	5.45
Metric Tons Consumed	187	597	63	128
Metric Tons Reported Seized	43.2	43.2	8.5	8.5
Metric Tons Manufactured	**230**	**640**	**72**	**137**
Intercepted (%)	19	7	12	6

Source: UNODC 2009c, 116.

combined with another chemical, results in a new product. The process of making methamphetamine starts with the precursor (ephedrine or pseudoephedrine), and other chemicals are added to produce the drug. Amphetamine manufacture takes place mostly in Europe, and ecstasy is, for the most part, manufactured in North America, Western Europe, and Oceania (UNODC 2008).

Consumption

Illicit drug use is difficult to assess accurately. This is particularly so for ATSs because markets appear and expand quickly, there is general confusion about what users actually consume, and there are limitations on reporting information. The number of ATS users is very uncertain; however, it has been reported that in 2007 there were between 16 and 51 million people aged 15–64 who consumed amphetamines-group substances (annual prevalence 0.4 to 1.2 percent). Ecstasy-group users numbered between 12 and 24 million worldwide (annual prevalence between 0.3 and 0.5 percent) (UNODC 2009c, 144).

At least half of the world's amphetamine users are in East and Southeast Asia, and most are methamphetamine users. The total number of amphetamine users in North America is estimated at around 3.8 million people, or 15 percent of global users. Europe accounts for about 10 percent of all users or 2.7 million people (see Figure 5.2).

Prevalence data from the 2009 National Survey on Drug Use and Health for persons aged 12 years or older show that there were 529,000 (0.2 percent) current users of methamphetamine and 760,000 (0.3 percent) of ecstasy (SAMHSA 2010). Prevalence data from 2008 show there were 314,000 (0.1 percent) current users of methamphetamine and 555,000 (0.2 percent) of ecstasy (SAMHSA 2009). Overall, there was an increase of current users of methamphetamine and ecstasy from 2008 to 2009. From 2002 to 2008, rates of current use of ecstasy, stimulants, and methamphetamine declined among youths aged 12 to 17 and young adults aged 18 to 25. For adults aged 25 or older, rates stayed steady. The rate of methamphetamine use tends to be similar for males and females.

According to the U.S. National Drug Intelligence Center, despite the decrease in number of amphetamine and methamphetamine users in the United States, "...methamphetamine production on the part of Mexican DTOs (i.e., drug trafficking organizations) in South American countries will likely continue in the near term, facilitating both an increase in methamphetamine production in Mexico and [its] subsequent flow...into the United States" (NDIC 2008).

References

Clines, F. X. 2001. "Kentucky Journal; Fighting Appalachia's Top Cash Crop, Marijuana." *New York Times*. Available at: http://www.nytimes.com/2001/02/28/us/kentucky-journal-fighting-appalachia-s-top-cash-crop-marijuana.html. Accessed October 25, 2009.

CNN. 2009. "Cocaine Seized on Submarine Near Guatemala." CNN Wire. October 22. Available at: http://cnnwire.blogs.cnn.com/2009/10/22/cocaine-seized-on-submarine-near-guatemala. Accessed October 23, 2009.

Costa, A. N. 2008. The 51st Session of the Commission on Narcotic Drugs. Available at: http://www.unodc.org/unodc/en/about-unodc/speeches/2008-03-10.html. Accessed September 7, 2010.

Kazancigil, A., and C. Milani. 2002. *Globalisation, Drugs and Criminalisation. Final Research Report on Brazil, China, India and Mexico*. New York: United Nations Office for Drug Control and Crime Prevention.

National Drug Intelligence Center (NDIC). 2008. *National Drug Threat Assessment 2009*. Available at: http://www.usdoj.gov/ndic/pubs31/31379/cocaine.htm#Top. Accessed September 23, 2009.

National Institute on Drug Abuse (NIDA). 1996. *Epidemiologic Trends in Drug Abuse,* vol. 1. *Highlights and Executive Summary*. Rockville, Md.: National Institutes of Health.

National Institute on Drug Abuse (NIDA). 2001. *Epidemiologic Trends in Drug Abuse,* vol. 1. *Highlights and Executive Summary*. Rockville, Md.: National Institutes of Health.

RAND Corporation. 2009. *Assessing Changes in Global Drug Problems, 1998–2007: Main Report*. Available at: http://www.rand.org/pubs/technical_reports/2009/RAND_TR704.pdf. Accessed June 7, 2009.

Schweich, T. 2008. "Is Afghanistan a Narco-State?" *New York Times Magazine*. July 27. Available at: http://www.nytimes.com/2008/07/27/magazine/27AFGHAN-t.html?ex=1217822400&en=b293a2810d8ad3ff&ei=5070&emc=eta1. Accessed June 7, 2009.

Substance Abuse and Mental Health Services Administration (SAMHSA). 2009. *Results from the 2008 National Survey on Drug Use and Health: National Findings*. Available at: http://www.oas.samhsa.gov/NSDUH/2k8NSDUH/2k8results.cfm#Ch2. Accessed September 7, 2010.

Substance Abuse and Mental Health Services Administration (SAMHSA). 2010. *Results from the 2009 National Survey on Drug Use and Health: National Findings*. Available at: http://www.drugabusestatistics.samhsa.gov/NSDUH/2k9NSDUH/2k9Results.htm. Accessed October 1, 2010.

United Nations. 1998. Guiding Principles of Drug Demand Reduction and Measures to Enhance International Cooperation to Counter the World Drug Problem. Special Session of the General Assembly Devoted to Countering the World Drug Problem Together, Political Declaration. Available at: http://www.unodc.org/pdf/report_1999–01–01_1.pdf. Accessed September 7, 2010.

United Nations Office for Drug Control and Crime Prevention (UNODCCP). 2002. *Global Illicit Drug Trends*. Available at: http://www.unodc.org/pdf/report_2002–06–26_1/report_2002–06–26_1.pdf. Accessed June 7, 2009.

United Nations Office on Drugs and Crime (UNODC). 2008. *2008 World Drug Report*. Available at: http://www.unodc.org/unodc/en/data-and-analysis/WDR-2008.html. Accessed June 7, 2009.

United Nations Office on Drugs and Crime (UNODC). 2009a. *Addiction, Crime and Insurgency: The Transnational Threat of Afghan Opium*. Available at: http://www.unodc.org/unodc/en/data-and-analysis/addiction-crime-and-insurgency.html. Accessed October 22, 2009.

United Nations Office on Drugs and Crime (UNODC). 2009b. *Afghan Opium Survey: Export Value of Afghan Opium is Falling*. Available at: http://www.unodc.org/unodc/en/frontpage/2009/December/export-value-of-afghan-opium-is-falling.html. Accessed December 19, 2009.

United Nations Office on Drugs and Crime (UNODC). 2009c. *World Drug Report 2009*. Available at: http://www.unodc.org/unodc/en/data-and-analysis/WDR-2009.html. Accessed September 7, 2009.

U.S. Office of International Information Agency (USIA). 1992. *Consequences of the Illegal Drug Trade: The Negative Economic, Political, and Social Effects of Cocaine in Latin America*. Washington, D.C.: USIA.

ADDITIONAL READINGS

Clawson, P., and L. Resselaer. n.d. *Consequences of the Illegal Drug Trade: The Negative Economic, Political and Social Effects of Cocaine on Latin America*. Washington, D.C.: U.S. Department of State, 2001.

European Monitoring Centre for Drugs and Drug Addiction. 2000. *Annual Report on the State of the Drug Problem in the European Union*. Available at: http://www.emcdda.europa.eu/html.cfm/index37279EN.html. Accessed October 23, 2009.

International Narcotics Control Board. 2010. *Report of the International Narcotics Control Board for 2009*. New York: United Nations.

Isralowitz, R. 2002. *Drug Use, Policy and Management*. Westport, Conn.: Auburn House.

National Institute on Drug Abuse (NIDA). 2000. *Epidemiologic Trends in Drug Abuse*, vol. 1. *Highlights and Executive Summary*. Rockville, Md.: National Institutes of Health.

Schlosser, E. 1997. "More Reefer Madness." *Atlantic* online (April). Available at: http://www.theatlantic.com/issues/97apr/reef.htm. Accessed October 25, 2009.

U.S. Department of Health and Human Services (DHHS). 2001. *Summary of Findings from the 2000 National Household Survey on Drug Abuse*. Rockville, Md.: Substance Abuse Mental Health Services Administration.

CHAPTER 6

People at Risk: Brief Profiles

Illicit drugs affect all groups of people. Among those at high risk of negative consequences from illicit drugs are children and youth, women, older adults, and racial and ethnic minority groups. The following information provides insight into each group.

CHILDREN AND YOUTH

Nearly all illicit drug use (e.g., marijuana/hashish, cocaine and crack, inhalants, hallucinogens, heroin, and prescription-type drugs used nonmedically) can be traced back to preadolescent and adolescent years. Generally, if a person has not begun to use illicit drugs during this period, the chances are that he or she never will. Among those who do use, school problems are likely to occur as a result, including low attendance rates, poor academic performance, dropping out, or expulsion. Other problems include delinquency, crime, risky sexual activities, and use of more dangerous drugs. Illicit drug use among youth is also related to higher death rates resulting from car accidents, suicide, homicide, and illness. Finally, many mental health problems among youth, including depression, anxiety, paranoia, hallucinations, developmental lags, delusions, and mood disturbances, may be linked to illicit drug use.

Trends: United States

The following information has been drawn from national and international sources including the U.S. Substance Abuse Mental Health Services Administration (SAMHSA), the Centers for Disease Control and Prevention (CDC), the World Health Organization (WHO), and the European Monitoring Centre for Drugs and Drug Addiction (EMCDDA).

A primary source of information on the use of illicit drugs, alcohol and tobacco in the United States is the annual National Survey on Drug Use and Health: National Findings (NSDUH) sponsored by the SAMHSA. The survey is conducted with a civilian, noninstitutionalized population aged 12 or older. Following are highlights of illicit drug use among youths from NSDUH (2009; 2010) and other sources:

- Among youths aged 12 to 17, about 9 percent reported being current (i.e., past month) illicit drug users. Most illicit drug use involves marijuana and nonmedical use of prescription-type psychotherapeutics followed by the use of inhalants, hallucinogens, and cocaine.
- Rates of current illicit drug use tend to be stable for all drugs except hallucinogens and nonmedical use of psychotherapeutics.
- Approximately one-tenth of U.S. youths aged 12 to 17 reported using nonprescribed pain relievers at least once in their lifetime. These youths were significantly more likely than those who did not use nonprescribed pain relievers to also report illicit drug use. For example, 49 percent of youths who used nonprescribed pain relievers also reported using two or more illicit drugs at least once in their lifetime, compared to 4 percent of youths who did not use nonprescribed pain relievers. Previous research has found a similar relationship between nonmedical use of prescription stimulants and use of other illicit drugs (Wu, Pilowsky, and Patkar 2008). Figure 6.1 provides patterns of past-month use of selected illicit drugs.

A major source of information about the behaviors, attitudes, and values of American high school and college students and young adults is Monitoring the Future (MTF), a report conducted by Institute of Survey Research at the University of Michigan with funds from the National Institute on Drug Abuse. Each year, approximately 50,000 high school students in the 8th, 10th, and 12th grades are surveyed (12th graders since 1975, and 8th and 10th graders since 1991). Recent MTF (2010) results for all grade levels combined show the following:

- Use of amphetamines, methamphetamine, and crystal meth has fallen. Also, there has been a decline in Ritalin use, an amphetamine drug prescribed to treat attention deficit hyperactivity disorder. For example, the number of high school students reporting past year use (2009) of amphetamines was 5.9 percent compared to 10.4 percent in 1996; methamphetamine use was 1.3 percent compared to 4.1 percent

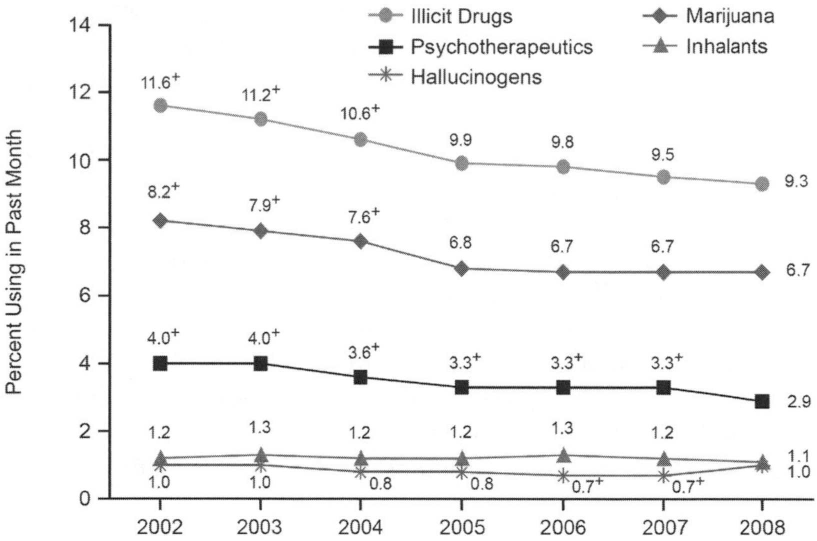

Figure 6.1 Past-month use of selected illicit drugs among youths aged 12 to 17 years, 2002–2008.

Source: SAMHSA 2009b.

in 1999; and Ritalin was 2.5 percent compared to 4.2 percent in 2002 when it was first measured.

- Marijuana remained the most widely used illicit drug. Marijuana use peaked in 1997 (30.1 percent) and since then annual prevalence has been in a gradual and steady decline; however, this pattern may be ending. In 2009 it was 22.9 percent, marking a gradual increase for the past two years with the key belief that the degree of risk with its use has declined.
- Anabolic steroids, primarily used by male teen students, evidenced a sharp increase in use in the late 1990s, peaking in 2000 at 2 percent. Since then, the annual prevalence rate has dropped by 50 percent to 1 percent for all grade levels. Lloyd Johnston, the lead research scientist for the MTF survey, has noted that a number of states and schools are considering implementing expensive programs to test student athletes for anabolic steroid use as a deterrent, despite the fact that the problem has diminished sharply.
- LSD, hallucinogens, ecstasy, and most of the prescription psychoactive drugs used outside of medical supervision, including sedatives (barbiturates), tranquilizers, and narcotics like heroin, OxyContin, and Vicodin tend to be holding steady in terms of patterns of use.

- Cocaine and crack use peaked among teens in the late 1990s, declined for a year or two, and has held relatively level in recent years. Annual cocaine and crack prevalence rates in 2009 were 2.5 and 1.2 percent, respectively.
- Most illicit drugs have shown considerable declines in use since the late 1990s. This is not the case, however, for most prescription drugs, with the notable exception of amphetamines. As a result, nonmedical use of prescription drugs has become a relatively more important part of the nation's illicit drug use problem.
- Over-the-counter cough and cold medications are sometimes taken for the purpose of getting high. Most of the drugs abused in this way contain the cough suppressant dextromethorphan as an active ingredient. It appears that attempts to discourage misuse of dextromethorphan have proven somewhat, but not entirely, successful.

Illicit Drug Use and Violence

Research suggests that youth violence and youth drug use are closely related. Getting into fights at school or work and involvement in group-against-group fights are more common among drug users. Youths aged 12 to 17, for example, are twice as likely to have engaged in violent behavior if they had used an illicit drug in the previous year (see Figure 6.2). Furthermore, the likelihood of engaging in violent behavior increases with the number of drugs used.

The national Youth Risk Behavior Survey (YRBS), conducted by the CDC, monitors health risk behaviors that contribute to the leading causes of death, disability, and social problems among youth and adults in the United States. The national YRBS is conducted every two years and provides information about illicit drug use among 9th- through 12th-grade students in public and private schools throughout the United States. Table 6.1 reflects patterns (in percentages) of illicit drug use among school age youth since 1991.

International Patterns

Since the 1960s, an increasing number of young people have been experimenting with drugs to the point where illicit drug use has become a serious problem in many countries. Cannabis is the primary illicit drug consumed in the European Union, and there has been a significant rise in use since the 1990s. Cannabis use among youth is of concern for a number of reasons, including health and legal problems and increased risk of psychosocial difficulties. For many people, cannabis use is an adolescent phenomenon that is unrelated to adult drug use; however, others

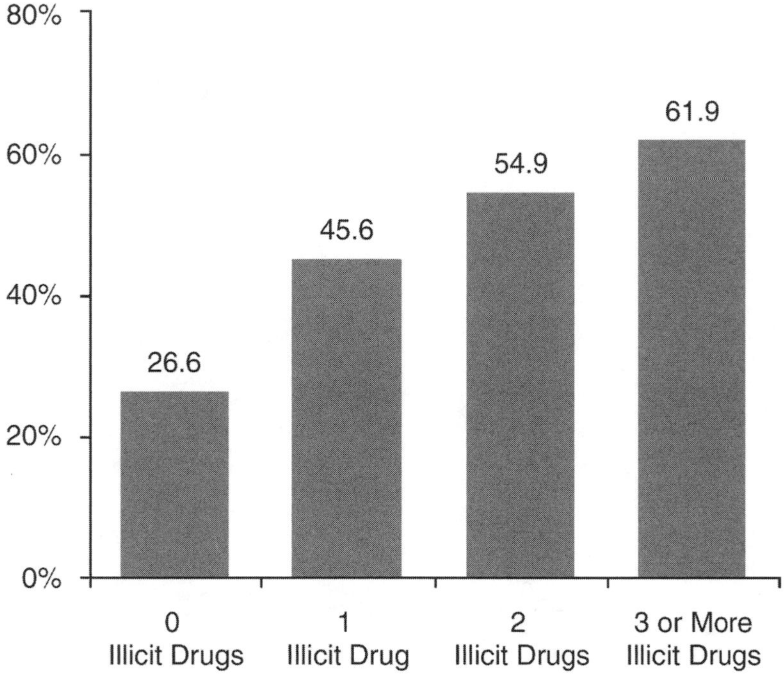

Figure 6.2 Percentages of youths aged 12 to 17 years who engaged in past-year violent behavior, by number of illicit drugs used in the past year, 2002, 2003, and 2004.

Source: SAMHSA 2006.

have reported that early cannabis use is predictive of later problematic psychosocial adjustment and an increased risk of cannabis dependence in adulthood.

According to the United Nations Commission on Narcotics, the drug prevalence rates among youth in many countries are as much as three or four times higher than for the general population. Patterns and trends in drug abuse among young people differ from region to region; however, in many countries, girls are as likely as boys to have used cannabis in the past 30 days. Young people in the United States, Canada, and Spain have the highest rates of cannabis use—generally 12–15 percent of the youth (WHO 2008). Amphetamine-type stimulant (ATS) abuse is widespread in Asia. And there are big variations in the prevalence of cocaine abuse. In Western Europe, for example, there have been increases in cocaine abuse, though at levels considerably lower than those in the United States. Injection of heroin has decreased dramatically in developed countries, but

Table 6.1 Trends in Prevalence of Marijuana, Cocaine, and Other Illegal Drug Use National YRBS: 1991–2009.

The national Youth Risk Behavior Survey (YRBS) monitors priority health risk behaviors that contribute to the leading causes of death, disability, and social problems among youth and adults in the United States. The national YRBS is conducted every two years during the spring semester and provides data representative of 9th through 12th grade students in public and private schools throughout the United States.

1991	1993	1995	1997	1999	2001	2003	2005	2007	2009	Changes from 1991–2009[1]	Change from 2007–2009[2]
Ever used marijuana one or more times (during their life)											
31.3 (28.4–34.4)[3]	32.8 (29.6–36.2)	42.4 (39.4–45.5)	47.1 (44.1–50.1)	47.2 (44.7–49.7)	42.4 (40.5–44.3)	40.2 (37.4–43.1)	38.4 (35.9–41.0)	38.1 (35.5–40.7)	36.8 (34.8–38.8)	Increased, 1991–1999 Decreased, 1999–2009	No change
Used marijuana one or more times (during the 30 days before the survey)											
14.7 (12.6–17.0)	17.7 (15.3–20.3)	25.3 (23.5–27.3)	26.2 (24.0–28.5)	26.7 (24.2–29.4)	23.9 (22.3–25.5)	22.4 (20.2–24.6)	20.2 (18.6–22.0)	19.7 (17.8–21.8)	20.8 (19.4–22.3)	Increased, 1991–1999 Decreased, 1999–2009	No change
Ever used any form of cocaine one or more times (for example, powder, crack, or freebase, during their life)											
5.9 (5.1–6.9)	4.9 (4.1–5.8)	7.0 (5.9–8.3)	8.2 (7.2–9.4)	9.5 (8.2–11.1)	9.4 (8.2–10.7)	8.7 (7.6–9.9)	7.6 (6.7–8.7)	7.2 (6.2–8.2)	6.4 (5.7–7.1)	Increased, 1991–1999 Decreased, 1999–2009	No change
Ever used methamphetamines one or more times (also called "speed", "crystal", "crank", or "ice", during their life)											
NA[4]	NA	NA	NA	9.1 (7.9–10.5)	9.8 (8.3–11.5)	7.6 (6.7–8.7)	6.2 (5.3–7.2)	4.4 (3.7–5.3)	4.1 (3.6–4.6)	No change, 1999–2001 Decreased, 2001–2009	No change

Ever sniffed glue, breathed the contents of aerosol spray cans, or inhaled any paints or sprays to get high one or more times (during their **life)**											
NA	NA	20.3 (18.3–22.5)	16.0 (14.7–17.3)	14.6 (12.9–16.5)	14.7 (13.1–16.6)	12.1 (10.9–13.4)	12.4 (11.1–13.8)	13.3 (12.1–14.6)	11.7 (10.6–12.8)	Decreased, 1995–2003 No change, 2003–2009	Decreased
Ever took steroid pills or shots without a doctor's prescription one or more times (during their life)											
2.7 (2.3–3.2)	2.2 (1.7–2.8)	3.7 (3.1–4.3)	3.1 (2.7–3.6)	3.7 (3.1–4.5)	5.0 (4.4–5.5)	6.1 (4.7–7.8)	4.0 (3.5–4.6)	3.9 (3.4–4.6)	3.3 (2.9–3.8)	Increased, 1991–2003 Decreased, 2003–2009	No change
Offered, sold or given an illegal drug by someone on school property (during the 12 months before the survey)											
NA	24.0 (21.4–26.8)	32.1 (29.1–35.3)	31.7 (29.9–33.5)	30.2 (27.8–32.7)	28.5 (26.5–30.6)	28.7 (24.9–32.8)	25.4 (23.3–27.6)	22.3 (20.3–24.4)	22.7 (20.7–24.9)	Increased 1993–1995 Decreased 1995–2009	No change

Source: Centers for Disease Control and Prevention 2010.

1. Based on trend analyses using a logistic regression model controlling for sex, race/ethnicity, and grade.

2. Based on t-test analyses, $p < 0.05$.

3. 95 percent confidence interval.

4. Not available.

is increasing among youth in Eastern Europe, while there are signs of a rise in abuse of smoking heroin in the United States. Abuse of inhalants, which are not under international control, is common, and remains a serious problem among children and young people in many countries (Family Health International 2008).

WOMEN

Although considerable progress has been made toward understanding illicit drug use, the problem has been sorely neglected in women. Men and women use drugs for different reasons. Females are more vulnerable to abuse and addiction because they become more dependent on drugs, such as crack cocaine, faster and suffer the consequences sooner than males.

Women often start using harmful drugs because of a stressful event. Studies show that women who abuse drugs often have health and mental problems, including those related to codependency, a history of parental alcohol and drug abuse, incest, and physical and sexual abuse (NIDA 2009). Socioeconomic factors are also related either directly or indirectly to drug abuse by women.

Women tend to begin abusing drugs later than men, and they are more likely to have a coexisting psychiatric problem, such as depression; more likely to report a greater history of suicide attempts; and, tend to be more hostile. Many women report that their drug-using male sex partners initiated them into drug abuse. In addition, drug-dependent women have great difficulty abstaining from drugs when the lifestyle of their male partner is one that supports drug use.

Many drug-using women do not seek treatment because they fear not being able to take care of or keep their children, reprisal from their spouses or boyfriends, and punishment from authorities in the community. Among those in need of treatment, many are faced with addressing a range of issues, including living with an alcoholic or addicted male partner, a lack of education, limited job experience, low self-esteem, and a lack of assertiveness skills, all of which make it difficult for them to manage the complex treatment and assistance network (Straussner and Brown 2002).

Trends

In 2008, the rate of current illicit drug use among persons age 12 years or older was lower for females than for males (6.3 percent versus 9.9 percent, respectively). Females were less likely to be current marijuana users (4.4 versus 7.9 percent); however, the nonmedical use of psychotherapeutic drugs was similar among females (2.4 percent) and males (2.6 percent).

In many developed countries, drug abuse is no longer a predominately male activity. In European countries, it has been reported that understanding drug use by women is a critical requirement for effective prevention and treatment responses to their needs. Following are key questions and issues related to drug abuse in Europe (ECAD 2006; EMCDDA 2006):

- *Is the gender gap in drug use narrowing?* Historically, prevalence rates of drug use among men have been considerably higher than those among women. Although this remains the case, surveys show that prevalence estimates for drug use are now more similar for male and female youths than for adults. This suggests a narrowing of the gender gap among the younger generations, which may result in an increase in the overall levels of prevalence in the future. Indeed, in some European Union countries females now equal males in their use of illicit drugs, and in most countries females surpass males in their misuse of tranquillizers and sedative drugs. As with their male counterparts, cannabis remains the illicit drug most widely used by European women but prevalence varies greatly between countries.
- *Barriers to treatment access.* The lack of social and economic support and childcare obligations have been identified as factors that can inhibit women from making use of drug treatment services. Also, women may be disinclined to enter inpatient treatment services, where they often represent an even smaller minority of clients than they do in outpatient services.
- *Low-threshold facilities for women.* Low-threshold agencies (i.e., agencies or services that help drug addicts with daily survival and help avoid their further deterioration) are available in a number of countries. They usually offer outreach, information, and advice, particularly about safe sex; provide sterile injecting equipment, condoms, and lubricants; and provide referrals to further health, social, and treatment services.
- *Interventions for pregnant women.* Outpatient and low-threshold facilities increasingly provide basic medical care, sexual health care, contraception advice, free infectious disease testing and treatment, and pregnancy tests. Pregnant drug users are defined as a priority group and the staff help them to jump the drug treatment queue.

Older Adults

Illegal drug use among older people is a concern because of the growing number with a history of such behavior. It is estimated that the population of adults older than 50 years with drug use and abuse problems will increase from 2.5 million in 1999 to 5 million in 2020, doubling the substance abuse treatment services needed for this population (Gfroerer et al. 2002; EMCDDA 2008; SAMHSA 2010).

In 2008, an estimated 4.3 million adults age 50 or older (4.7 percent of adults in that age range) had used an illicit drug in the past year. Marijuana use was more common than nonmedical use of prescription-type drugs for those up to age 59; however, for those aged 65 and older, nonmedical use of prescription-type drugs was more common. These patterns and trends may be the result of an aging baby boom cohort, whose lifetime rates of illicit drug use are higher than those of older cohorts. Illicit drug use (e.g., marijuana) is primarily a male problem; however, the rate of nonmedical use of prescription-type drugs tends to be greater among older women than older men especially for those aged 60 to 64 (SAMHSA 2009a).

Illicit drug use is also a problem among persons with co-occurring mental health problems and regular users of recreational drugs who may experience more complications with aging. Additional factors to consider are that drugs in older adults metabolize more slowly and many stimulants lead to changes in brain function that may have long-term effects, including impairments associated with aging. Relatively little is known about the treatment of drug use in older adults. However, older patients do well with treatment programs and can achieve satisfactory treatment outcomes.

Older adults are the biggest consumers of prescription and over-the-counter medications; and, they are vulnerable to misuse and the medication's adverse effects (Qato et al. 2008). This is a major public health problem that leads to mortality, morbidity, and related health costs. Studies have documented the level of potentially inappropriate medication among nursing home residents and elderly people in community-based care facilities (Isralowitz, Reznik, and Borkin 2006; Topinkova et al. 2005; Spore et al. 1995).

Key signals related to nonmedical use of prescription drugs are memory trouble after taking medicine; loss of coordination (walking unsteadily, frequent falls); changes in sleeping habits; unexplained bruises; being unsure of oneself; irritability, sadness, and depression; unexplained chronic pain; changes in eating habits; the desire to stay alone a lot of the time; failure to wash or keep clean; impaired, slurred speech and difficulty finishing sentences; difficulty concentrating; difficulty staying in touch with family or friends; and lack of interest in usual activities (SAMHSA 2004). Reasons for misuse of medications include difficulties reading and following prescriptions, cognitive deficits, cost, and complexity of drug treatment. Misuse and abuse have been linked to genetics, stress, depression, comorbidities, metabolism, and dosage.

Racial and Ethnic Minorities

The United States is in demographic transition—the whites are a declining percentage of the population, and the number of racial/ethnic minorities is on the rise. Considerable attention is being given to epidemiologic data about illicit drug use to understand the extent of the problem for these populations. For example, patterns of drug use in the country are monitored by government supported surveillance methods including the NSDUH; the Drug Abuse Warning Network, a national survey of hospital emergency departments; the previously described MTF, a study of the behaviors, attitudes, and values of American secondary school students, college students, and young adults; and the National Institute of Drug Abuse's (NIDA) Community Epidemiology Work Group, a network composed of researchers from major metropolitan areas of the United States and selected foreign countries that meet semiannually to discuss the current epidemiology of drug abuse.

Definition of Race and Ethnicity

Any understanding of illegal drug use and racial/ethnic minorities must address definitions of race and ethnicity that tend to vary by investigation. For some, race is a mere social construct, and differences among people depend more on perceptions and less on fundamental biological differences (Condit, Condit, and Achter 2001). The benchmark for defining race and ethnicity in the United States is a federal Office of Management and Budget announcement issued in October 1997. The 2008 National Survey on Drug Use and Health (NSDUH) uses the following definition for race and ethnicity (SAMHSA 2009b):

> Race/ethnicity is used to refer to the respondent's self-classification of racial and ethnic origin and identification. For Hispanic origin, respondents were asked, "Are you of Hispanic, Latino, or Spanish origin or descent?" For race, respondents were asked, "Which of these groups best describes you?" Response alternatives were (1) white, (2) black/African American, (3) American Indian or Alaska Native, (4) Native Hawaiian, (5) Other Pacific

Islander, (6) Asian, and (7) Other. Categories for a combined race/ethnicity variable included Hispanic; non-Hispanic groups where respondents indicated only one race (white, black, American Indian or Alaska Native, Native Hawaiian or Other Pacific Islander, Asian); and non-Hispanic groups where respondents reported two or more races. These categories are based on classifications developed by the U.S. Census Bureau.

Among racial/ethnic groups, the rate of current illicit drug use was the lowest among Asians (3.6 percent) and highest for those with two or more races (14.7 percent). Figure 6.3 shows past-month illicit drug use for all groups.

The following information is summarized from the NIDA (2003) report *Drug Use Among Racial and Ethnic Minorities* except where noted.

American Indians/Alaska Natives

Serious concern exists that American Indian/Alaska Native populations have not been well represented in national statistics and surveillance activities for drug involvement (e.g., too few American Indian/Alaska Native participants in the surveys)...and some research indicates more excessive

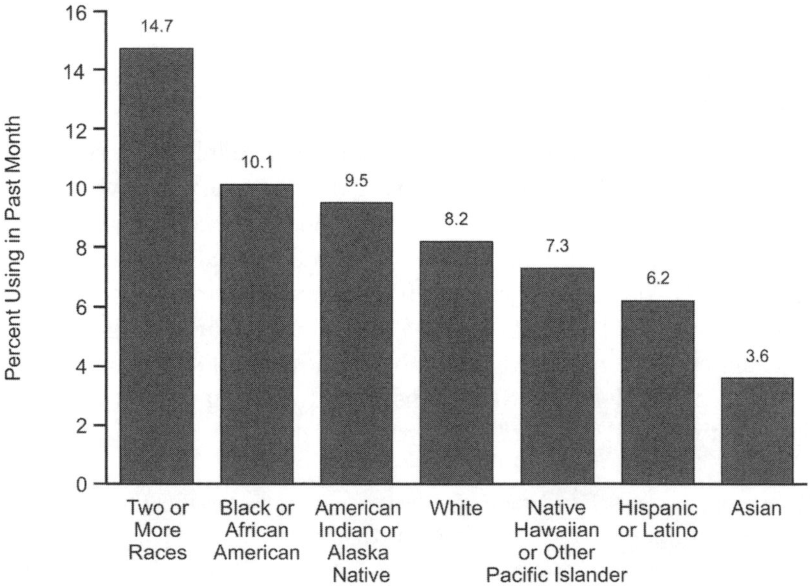

Figure 6.3 Past-month illicit drug use among persons aged 12 years or older, by race/ethnicity, 2008.

Source: SAMHSA 2009b.

drinking and illegal drug use among American Indians and Alaska Natives than among most, if not all, other racial/ethnic minority groups.

Asian/Pacific Islanders

Asian/Pacific Islanders comprise more than 60 separate racial/ethnic groups and subgroups that are heterogeneous... [Slightly] more than 6 percent of Americans age 12 and older are current illegal drug users... For Asian/Pacific Islanders... Chinese Americans... Asian Indian Americans... Filipino Americans... Vietnamese Americans... and Japanese Americans [the rate of illicit drug use tends to be lower].

African Americans

National statistics tend to convey information about African Americans in a single grouped category, despite what we know of the considerable heterogeneity within African American communities... Some studies have given the impression that African Americans who use alcohol and other drugs experience higher rates of drug-related health problems than do users from other ethnic groups. Other studies indicate that the estimated rate of transition from drug use to drug dependence is no greater for African Americans... There is some reason to believe that general impressions about African Americans and drug problems are based on partial evidence, traced back to racial profiling and other administrative practices that lead to overrepresentation of African Americans in criminal justice statistics and in public drug treatment programs where admissions draw heavily on referrals from the courts (e.g., see Blumstein and Beck 1999)... "African American students have substantially lower rates of use of most licit and illicit drugs than do Whites." (Johnston et al. 2010)

Hispanics

Studies of Hispanic young people indicate a greater tendency toward higher prevalence of several forms of drug involvement among Hispanic adolescents than among their counterparts in the non-Hispanic, African American, and White segments of the population... "Hispanics do have the highest reported rates of use for some drugs in 12th grade—crack, methamphetamine, and crystal methamphetamine. In 8th grade, they tend to come out highest among the racial/ethnic groups on nearly all types of drugs." (Johnston et al. 2010)

Understanding which sociodemographic factors (e.g., region, population density, language of interview, family income, health insurance coverage, receipt of welfare, educational attainment, school dropout status, marital status, employment status, and number of children) are associated with racial/ethnic differences in illicit drug use is difficult. Moreover, regardless of racial/ethnic subgroup, adolescents who dropped out of school or who reside in households with only one biological parent have a relatively high prevalence of past-year use of cigarettes, alcohol, and illicit drugs (SAMHSA 2008).

References

Blumstein, A., and A. Beck. 1999. "Population Growth in U.S. Prisons, 1980–1996." In *Prisons: Crime and Justice, A Review of Research*, vol. 26, ed. M. Tonry and J. Petersilia. Chicago, Ill.: University of Chicago Press.

Centers for Disease Control and Prevention. 2010. Trends in Prevalence of Marijuana, Cocaine, and Other Illegal Drug Use. National YRBS: 1991–2009. Available at: http://www.cdc.gov/healthyyouth/yrbs/pdf/us_drug_trend_yrbs.pdf. Accessed October 2, 2010.

Condit, C., D. Condit, and P. Achter. 2001. "Human Equality, Affirmative Action, and Genetic Models of Human Variation." *Rhetoric and Public Affairs* 4 (1): 85–108.

European Cities Against Drugs (ECAD). 2006. "EMCDDA: Women and Drug Use in Europe." *ECAD Newsletter*. Available at: http://www.ecad.net/nyh6/news88_89en.pdf. Accessed September 10, 2010.

European Monitoring Centre for Drugs and Drug Addiction (EMCDDA). 2006. *Annual Report 2006*. Available at: http://ar2006.emcdda.europa.eu/download/ar2006-en.pdf. Accessed September 10, 2010.

European Monitoring Centre for Drugs and Drug Addiction (EMCDDA). 2008. "Substance Use Among Older Adults: A Neglected Problem." *Drugs in Focus* 18 (1). Available at: www.emcdda.europa.eu/attachements.cfm/att_50566_EN_TDAD08001ENC_web.pdf. Accessed September 10, 2010.

Family Health International. 2008. Youth and Injecting Drug Users. Available at: http://www.fhi.org/NR/rdonlyres/ewrxgzw2rkkxsgb3i2x5dhfo52ffo7xvwad7nodvndoop2fwhht5loxodtkayqyxjzgb2sg2do6m6j/YL26e1.pdf. Accessed September 9, 2010.

Gfroerer, J., M. Penne, M. Pemberton, and R. Folson Jr. 2002. "The Aging Baby Boom Cohort and Future Prevalence of Substance Abuse." In *Substance Use by Older Adults: Estimates of Future Impact on the Treatment System*. OAS Analytic Series A-21, DHHS Publication No. (SMA) 03-3763, Rockville, Md.: SAMHSA. Available at: http://www.drugabusestatistics.samhsa.gov/aging/chap5.htm. Accessed September 10, 2010.

Isralowitz, R., A. Reznik, and S. Borkin. 2006. "Late Life Benzodiazepine Use among Russian Speaking Immigrants in Israel." *Gerontologist* 46 (5): 677–79.

Johnston, L., P. O'Malley, J. Bachman, and J. Schulenberg. 2010. *Monitoring the Future: National Results on Adolescent Drug Use. Overview of Key Findings, 2007*. Available at: http://drugabuse.gov/PDF/overview2007.pdf. Accessed September 10, 2010.

Monitoring the Future (MTF). 2010. Overview of Key Findings 2009. Available at: http://monitoringthefuture.org/pubs/monographs/overview2009.pdf. Accessed September 9, 2010.

National Institute on Drug Abuse (NIDA). 2003. *Drug Use among Racial/Ethnic Minorities*, rev. ed. Available at: http://archives.drugabuse.gov/pubs/minorities. Accessed September 10, 2010.

National Institute on Drug Abuse (NIDA). 2009. "NIDA InfoFacts: Treatment Approaches for Drug Addiction." Available at: http://www.drugabuse.gov/infofacts/treatmeth.html. Accessed September 10, 2010.

Qato, D., G. Alexander, R. Conti, M. Johnson, P. Schumm, and S. Lindau. 2008. Use of Prescription and Over-the-counter Medications and Dietary Supplements Among Older Adults in the United States. *JAMA* 300 (24): 2867–78.

Spore, D., V. Mor, J. Hiris, E. Larrat, and C. Hawes. 1995. "Psychotropic Use among Older Residents of Board and Care Facilities. *Journal of the American Geriatrics Society* 43 (12): 1403–9.

Straussner, S., and S. Brown, eds. 2002. *The Handbook of Addiction Treatment for Women: Theory and Practice*. New York: Guilford Press.

Substance Abuse Mental Health Services Administration (SAMHSA). 2004. *As You Are…A Guide to Aging, Medicines and Alcohol.* Available at: http://asyouage.samhsa.gov/media/asyouage/asyouagebrochure01.pdf. Accessed September 10, 2010.

Substance Abuse Mental Health Services Administration (SAMHSA). 2006. "Youth Violence and Illicit Drug Use." *The NSDUH Report* 5. Available at: http://www.oas.samhsa.gov/2k6/youthViolence/youthViolence.htm. Accessed October 1, 2010.

Substance Abuse Mental Health Services Administration (SAMHSA). 2008. Prevalence of Substance Use among Racial and Ethnic Subgroups in the U.S. Available at: http://www.oas.samhsa.gov/NHSDA/ethnic/ethn1006.htm. Accessed September 10, 2010.

Substance Abuse Mental Health Services Administration (SAMHSA). 2009a. *Illicit Drug Use among Older Adults*. Available at: http://www.oas.samhsa.gov/2k9/168/168OlderAdults.htm. Accessed September 10, 2010.

Substance Abuse Mental Health Services Administration (SAMHSA). 2009b. *Results from the 2008 National Survey on Drug Use and Health: National Findings.* Available at: http://www.oas.samhsa.gov/nsduh/2k8nsduh/2k8Results.cfm#2.7. Accessed September 10, 2010.

Substance Abuse Mental Health Services Administration (SAMHSA). 2010. "Increasing Substance Abuse Levels among Older Adults Likely to Create Sharp Rise in Need for Treatment Services in Next Decade." Available at: http://samhsa.gov/newroom/advisories/1001073150. Accessed September 10, 2010.

Topinkova, F., G. Gambassi, H. Finne-Soveri, P. Jonsson, I. Carpenter, M. Schroll, G. Onder, L. Sorbye, C. Wagner, J. Reissigova, and R. Bernabei. 2005. "Use of Potentially Inappropriate Medication Use among Elderly Home Care Patients in Europe." *JAMA* 293 (11): 1348–58.

World Health Organization (WHO). 2008. *Inequalities in Young People's Health: HBSC International Report from the 2005/2006 Survey*. Available at: http://

www.euro.who.int/__data/assets/pdf_file/0005/53852/E91416.pdf. Accessed September 10, 2010.

Wu, L., D. Pilowsky, and A. Patkar. 2008. "Non-prescribed Use of Pain Relievers Among Adolescents in the United States." *Drug and Alcohol Dependence* 94 (1–3): 1–11.

Additional Readings

Center on Addiction and Substance Abuse at Columbia University (CASA). 2003. *The Formative Years: Pathways to Substance Abuse Among Girls and Young Women Ages 8–22*. Available at: http://www.casacolumbia.org/absolutenm/articlefiles/380-Formative_Years_Pathways_to_Substance_Abuse.pdf. Accessed September 10, 2010.

Child Trends Data Bank. 2008. Substance Free Youth. Available at: http://www.childtrendsdatabank.org/indicators/58IllicitDrugUse.cfm. Accessed September 10, 2010.

Curley, B. 2008. "Youth Use of Legal Drugs Eclipses Illicit-Drug Use, Annual Survey Reports." December 11. Join Together Online. Available at: http://www.jointogether.org/news/features/2008/youth-use-of-legal-drugs.html. Accessed September 10, 2010.

European Monitoring Centre for Drugs and Drug Addiction (EMCDDA). 2006. A Gender Perspective on Drug Use and Responding to Drug Problems. Available at: http://www.emcdda.europa.eu/attachements.cfm/att_37291_EN_sel2006_2-en.pdf. Accessed September 10, 2010.

European Monitoring Centre for Drugs and Drug Addiction (EMCDDA). 2008. Online Glossary. Available at: http://www.emcdda.europa.eu/publications/glossary. Accessed September 10, 2010.

Herd, D. 1989. "The Epidemiology of Drinking Patterns and Alcohol Related Problems among U.S. African Americans." In *Alcohol Use among U.S. Ethnic Minorities* (Research Monograph 18. DHHS Pub. No. [ADM] 89–1435), 3–50. Rockville, Md.: National Institute on Alcohol Abuse and Alcoholism.

Isralowitz, R., and A. Reznik. 2008. "Problem Severity Profiles of Substance Abusing Women in Therapeutic Treatment Facilities." *International Journal of Mental Health and Addiction* 7 (2): 368–75.

Leshner, A. 1998. "Foreword." In *Drug Addiction Research and the Health of Women*, ed. C. Wetherington and A. Roman (NIH Publication No. 98–4289). Bethesda, Md.: National Institutes of Health.

Longo, L., and B. Johnson. 2000. "Addiction: Part 1. Benzodiazepines—Side Effects, Abuse Risk and Alternatives." *American Family Physician* 61:2120–28.

Moos, R., P. Brennan, K. Schutte, and B. Moos. 2004. "High-risk Alcohol Consumption and Late-life Alcohol Use Problems." *American Journal of Public Health* 94 (11): 1985–91.

National Institute on Drug Abuse (NIDA). 1998. Drug Addiction Research and the Health of Women. Available at: http://archives.drugabuse.gov/WHGD/DARHW-download.html. Accessed September 10, 2010.

National Institute on Drug Abuse (NIDA). 2004. *Drug Abuse in the 21st Century: What Problems Lie Ahead for the Baby Boomers?* Available at: http://archives.drugabuse.gov/meetings/bbsr/prevalence.html. Accessed September 10, 2010.

National Institute on Drug Abuse (NIDA). 2008. Monitoring the Future, Overview of Key Findings, 2008. Available at: http://www.nida.nih.gov/PDF/overview2008.pdf. Accessed September 10, 2010.

National Institute on Drug Abuse (NIDA). 2009. "Teen Methamphetamine Use, Cigarette Smoking at Lowest Levels in NIDA's 2009 Monitoring the Future Survey." Available at: http://www.nih.gov/news/health/dec2009/nida-14.htm. Accessed September 10, 2010.

Office of National Drug Control Policy. n.d. "Women, Girls and Drugs: Facts and Figures." Available at: http://www.whitehousedrugpolicy.gov/drugfact/women/women_ff.html. Accessed September 10, 2010.

Roberts, M., M. King, J. Stokes, et al. 1998. "Medication Prescribing and Administration in Nursing Homes." *Age and Ageing* 27 (3): 385–92.

Simoni-Wastila, L. 2000. "The Use of Abusable Prescription Drugs: The Role of Gender." *Journal of Women's Health and Gender-Based Medicine* 9 (3): 289–97.

Simoni-Wastila, L. 2003. "Prescription Drug Nonmedical Use and Abuse in Older Women." National Institute of Drug Abuse. Available at: http://archives.drugabuse.gov/meetings/bbsr/prescription.html. Accessed September 10, 2010.

Substance Abuse Mental Health Services Administration (SAMHSA). 2001. *Summary of Findings from the 2000 National Household Survey on Drug Abuse* (DHHS Pub. No. [SMA] 01–3549). Rockville, Md.: SAMHSA. Available at: http://www.oas.samhsa.gov/NHSDA/2kNHSDA/2knhsda.htm. Accessed September 10, 2010.

Substance Abuse Mental Health Services Administration (SAMHSA). 2008. *Results from the 2007 National Survey on Drug Use and Health: National Findings.* Available at: http://www.oas.samhsa.gov/NSDUH/2k7NSDUH/2k7results.cfm. Accessed September 10, 2010.

Substance Abuse and Mental Health Services Administration (SAMHSA). 2010. *Results from the 2009 National Survey on Drug Use and Health: National Findings.* Available at: http://www.drugabusestatistics.samhsa.gov/NSDUH/2k9NSDUH/2k9Results.htm. Accessed October 1, 2010

United Nations Office on Drugs and Crime (UNODC). 2004. *Substance Abuse Treatment and Care for Women.* Available at: http://www.unodc.org/pdf/report_2004-08-30_1.pdf. Accessed September 10, 2010.

University of Michigan News Service. 2009. "Teen Marijuana Use Tilts Up, While Some Drugs Decline in Use." Available at: http://monitoringthefuture.org/pressreleases/09drugpr.pdf. Accessed September 10, 2010.

U.S. Bureau of the Census. 2000. *Projections of the Resident Population by Race, Hispanic Origin, and Nativity: Middle Series, 1999–2100.* Available at: http://www.census.gov/population/projections/nation/summary/np-t.txt. Accessed September 10, 2010.

CHAPTER 7

Key Issues and Controversies

Many illicit drug issues have generated concern and attention. In this chapter, controversies surrounding cannabis (marijuana and hashish), inhalants, crack cocaine, methamphetamine, hallucinogens (LSD and ecstasy), and prescription drugs are examined.

CANNABIS (MARIJUANA/HASHISH)

Cannabis, which includes marijuana and hashish, has generated more controversy and response to its impact on individual behavior and society than any other illegal drug in the United States. Information about cannabis, specifically marijuana, tends to be presented in ways that support the interests of those who advocate legal regulation of the drug because of its harmful effects or those who advocate legalization because of its helpful and benign characteristics.

General Background

According to the 2010 National Survey on Drug Use and Health, an estimated 16.7 million Americans aged 12 or older were current marijuana users. Marijuana was used by 76.6 percent of current illicit drug users and was the only drug used by 58 percent of them (SAMHSA 2010c). Marijuana is the leading U.S. cash crop, exceeding the value of corn and wheat combined (Gettman 2006). Among high school students the perceived availability of marijuana has remained high and steady despite a decades-long nationwide drug war. For the first time since the late 1970s and early 1980s, marijuana use has rivaled cigarette use among this population.

Legal and Policy Perspectives

Cannabis (i.e., marijuana and hashish) became a federally prohibited drug in 1937—a time when few Americans had ever heard about it. Federal law restricts its possession, use, purchase, sale, or cultivation. The Controlled Substances Act of 1970 classifies cannabis, like heroin, as a Schedule I drug, claiming it has a high potential for abuse and no acceptable medical purpose. A Supreme Court decision (*Gonzales v. Raich* 2005) allowed the federal government to ban cannabis use, even for medical purposes.

Under federal law, cultivation of even one marijuana plant is a felony, and lengthy mandatory minimum sentences apply to numerous marijuana-related offenses. For example, a person must serve a five-year mandatory sentence for a federal conviction of cultivating 100 marijuana plants. This is longer than the average sentences for auto theft and manslaughter. Civil forfeiture laws allow police to seize the money and property of suspected marijuana offenders—charges need not be filed. The claim is against property, not the defendant. The property owner must then prove that the property is "innocent." Enforcement abuses stemming from forfeiture laws abound (MPP 2008). Table 7.1 shows federal trafficking penalties for cannabis/marijuana (DEA 2010).

Nearly half (47 percent) of the total arrests for drug abuse violations in the United States are for marijuana sale/manufacturing and possession. In 2007, 51 percent of all drug possession violations were for marijuana, and 89 percent of all marijuana arrests were for possession only. Some states (e.g., Alaska, California, Colorado, New York, North Carolina, Maine, Minnesota, Mississippi, Nebraska, Ohio, and Oregon) have taken action to decriminalize and/or have asked law enforcement agencies to limit enforcement of cannabis laws. This action has reduced the number of simple-possession offenders sent to jail and saved enforcement costs. Small fines may be issued (similar to traffic tickets), but there is no arrest, incarceration, or criminal record. Presently, federal judicial decisions are moving toward favoring state law that permits marijuana's use, especially for medical purposes.

Facts and Arguments

For

There is no conclusive evidence that marijuana is causally linked to the subsequent use or abuse of other illicit drugs. The Institute of Medicine has characterized marijuana's role as a "gateway drug" as follows:

> Because it is the most widely used illicit drug, marijuana is predictably the first illicit drug most people encounter... [m]ost users of other illicit drugs

Table 7.1 Federal Trafficking Penalties for Cannabis/Marijuana

	Quantity	1st Offense	2nd Offense
Marijuana	1,000 kg or more mixture; or 1,000 or more plants.	Not less than 10 years, not more than life. If death or serious injury, not less than 20 years, not more than life. Fine not more than $4 million individual, $10 million other than individual.	Not less than 20 years, not more than life. If death or serious injury, then life. Fine not more than $8 million individual, $20 million other than individual.
Marijuana	100–999 kg mixture; or 100–999 plants.	Not less than 5 years, not more than 40 years. If death or serious injury, not less than 20 years, not more than life. Fine not more than $2 million individual, $5 million other than individual.	Not less than 10 years, not more than life. If death or serious injury, then life. Fine not more than $4 million individual, $10 million other than individual.
Marijuana Hashish Hashish Oil	50–99 kg mixture; 50–99 plants. More than 10 kg. More than 1 kg.	Not more than 20 years. If death or serious injury, not less than 20 years, not more than life. Fine $1 million individual, $5 million other than individual.	Not more than 30 years. If death or serious injury, then life. Fine $2 million individual, $10 million other than individual.
Marijuana Hashish Hashish Oil	Less than 50 kg mixture; 1–49 plants. 10 kg or less. 1 kg or less.	Not more than 5 years. Fine not more than $250,000 individual, $1 million other than individual.	Not more than 10 years. Fine $500,000 individual, $2 million other than individual.

Note: Includes hashish and hashish oil. Marijuana is a Schedule I controlled substance.

Source: DEA 2010.

> have used marijuana first. In fact, most drug users begin with alcohol and nicotine before marijuana—usually before they are of legal age... [In] the sense that marijuana use typically precedes rather than follows initiation of other illicit drug use, it is indeed a "gateway" drug. But because underage smoking and alcohol use typically precede marijuana use, marijuana is not the most common, and is rarely the first, "gateway" to illicit drug use. There is no conclusive evidence that the drug effects of marijuana are causally linked to the subsequent abuse of other illicit drugs. (Joy, Watson, and Benson 1999)

Commissioned by President Nixon, the National Commission on Marihuana and Drug Abuse stated that "marihuana's relative potential for harm to the vast majority of individual users and its actual impact on society does not justify a social policy designed to seek out and firmly punish those who use it." When examining the relationship between marijuana use and violent crime, it was concluded that, "rather than inducing violent or aggressive behavior through its purported effects of lowering inhibitions, weakening impulse control and heightening aggressive tendencies, marihuana was usually found to inhibit the expression of aggressive impulses by pacifying the user, interfering with muscular coordination, reducing psychomotor activities and generally producing states of drowsiness lethargy, timidity and passivity" (National Commission on Marihuana and Drug Abuse 1972).

A literature search and testimony of the nation's health officials reveals that there is little chance of overdose death from smoking marijuana. This is in marked contrast to other substances in common use, most notably alcohol and barbiturate sleeping pills. The World Health Organization (WHO) released a study in March 1998 stating that the public health risks from cannabis are much less serious than those associated with alcohol and tobacco use.

Since 1969, government-appointed commissions in the United States, Canada, England, Australia, and the Netherlands have concluded, after reviewing the scientific evidence, that the dangers of marijuana have been greatly exaggerated and urged lawmakers to drastically reduce or eliminate penalties for marijuana possession. In its 2002 final report on cannabis policy, the Canadian Senate's Special Committee on Illegal Drugs recommended that "the Government of Canada amend the Controlled Drugs and Substances Act to create a criminal exemption scheme. This report recommended conditions for obtaining licenses as well as for producing and selling cannabis; criminal penalties for illegal trafficking and export; and the preservation of criminal penalties for all activities falling outside the scope of the exception scheme" (Canada Special Senate Committee on Illegal Drugs 2002).

The Police Foundation of the United Kingdom stated

> that the present law on cannabis produces more harm than it prevents. It is very expensive of the time and resources of the criminal justice system and especially of the police. It inevitably bears more heavily on young people in the streets of inner cities, who are also more likely to be from minority ethnic communities, and as such is inimical to police-community relations. It criminalizes large numbers of otherwise law-abiding, mainly young, people to the detriment of their futures. It has become a proxy for the control of public order; and it inhibits accurate education about the relative risks of different drugs including the risks of cannabis itself. (Runciman 2000)

In 2002, the UK Home Secretary David Blunkett announced that "we must concentrate our efforts on the drugs that cause the most harm, while sending a credible message to young people. I will therefore ask Parliament to reclassify cannabis from Class B to Class C," which involves fewer penalties. In 2004, cannabis was reclassified as a Class C drug, a category that includes anabolic steroids and benzodiazepine. In January 2009, this action was reversed again to Class B because of uncertainty about the drug and its future impact on young people's mental health.

Against

Short-terms effects of marijuana use have been reported to include distortions of sight, sound, time, and touch; problems with memory and learning; poor coordination; difficulty with thinking and problem solving; increased heart rate; and reduced blood pressure. It can also produce anxiety, fear, distrust, or panic. High doses of marijuana can cause hallucinations, delusion, impaired memory, and disorientation. Regular use can cause respiratory problems, cough, phlegm, lung infections, and breathing difficulties. Children born to mothers who use marijuana during pregnancy exhibit some neurological development problems.

According to the federal Potency Monitoring Project, supported by the U.S. National Institute on Drug Administration (NIDA), the average quantity of THC, the psychoactive ingredient in marijuana, reached its highest level ever in 2009—10.1 percent (ONDCP 2009). In England, the Home Office reported the THC potency levels of cannabis in 2008 to be 8.4 percent to 16.2 percent, depending on the nature of the marijuana (British Home Office 2008).

In response to these levels, NIDA reported that the increases in marijuana potency are of concern because they increase the likelihood of acute toxicity, including mental impairment. Recent research shows that cannabis has a wide range of psychological and symptomatic effects that can induce psychotic symptoms and anxiety, and regular use is associated with cognitive impairments and an increased risk of schizophrenia, but these conclusions have been disputed.

Does marijuana have any medical value? The Institute of Medicine of the National Academy of Sciences is a private, nongovernment organization that does not receive direct federal appropriations for its work but conducts studies at the request of government agencies. In a comprehensive study on the health benefits of marijuana, it concluded that symptoms, if not diseases, can be relieved by marijuana, but for most patients there are more effective approved medicines. On the other hand, there are possible benefits from certain cannabinoids in combination with other drugs. Continued research to elaborate that potential and epidemiological studies to define risks from smoking marijuana are recommended (Mack and Joy 2000).

In considering whether marijuana harms anyone other than the person who smokes it, a Drug Enforcement Administration (DEA) fact sheet states that "marijuana affects many skills required for safe driving: alertness, the ability to concentrate, coordination, and reaction time. These effects can last up to 24 hours after smoking marijuana. Marijuana use can make it difficult to judge distances and react to signals and signs on the road," causing accidents and fatalities (DEA n.d.).

The DEA makes the following claims about the harms of marijuana:

- Marijuana is a dangerous, addictive drug that poses significant health threats to users.
- Marijuana has no medical value that can't be met more effectively by legal drugs.
- Marijuana users are far more likely to use other drugs like cocaine and heroin than non-marijuana users.
- Drug legalizers use "medical marijuana" as [a] red herring in [an] effort to advocate broader legalization of drug use (DEA n.d.).

Medical Marijuana

The cannabis plant has been used for medicinal purposes for thousands of years. Among its most commonly used purposes are in the treatment of nausea, vomiting, weight loss, and lack of appetite—symptoms associated with the treatment of cancer, acquired immunodeficiency syndrome

(AIDS), inflammatory bowel disease, and hepatitis. Thirteen states have approved the medical use of marijuana for qualified patients, though its use remains illegal under federal law. Intense debate has circled such medical uses of the drug. Supporters often point to FDA criteria for approving drugs, arguing that marijuana's medical benefits—including treatment of conditions ranging from AIDS to glaucoma, multiple sclerosis, and epilepsy—significantly outweigh any risks associated with its use. Many even argue that deaths associated with legal prescription drug use could be significantly reduced if medical marijuana were more widely available as an alternative. On the other side of the debate, many argue that marijuana use does indeed carry significant risks, including addiction, impaired driving, and injury to the lungs, immune system, and brain. Some also see marijuana as a gateway drug leading to more dangerous types of drug use or see its medical use as a first step toward legalization of the drug for recreational uses (ProCon.org 2009).

In addition to the 14 states and the District of Columbia that have made provisions for the medical use of marijuana (see Table 7.2), Arizona and Maryland have passed laws that are favorable to medical marijuana without actually legalizing its use.

Organizations that have endorsed medical access to marijuana include the American College of Physicians, Leukemia and Lymphoma Society, American Academy of Family Physicians, American Public Health Association, and British Medical Association. In November 2009, the American Medical Association (AMA) reversed its 72-year policy that marijuana be retained as a Schedule I substance (i.e., a drug or other substance that has a high potential for abuse, no accepted medical use, and a lack of accepted safety for use under medical supervision). Among the drugs included in this category are heroin, MDMA or ecstasy, and LSD. The AMA affirmed the therapeutic benefits of marijuana and called for further research (American Medical Association 2009).

In 2005, the U.S. Supreme Court ruled in *Raich v. Gonzales* that the federal government can prosecute medical marijuana patients even in states with laws permitting its use. In 2009, the Supreme Court refused to hear a legal challenge by San Diego County to overturn California's medical marijuana law permitting use. In a Justice Department memo to federal prosecutors in the states that allow the use of marijuana for medical purposes, the attorney general Eric Holder Jr. suggested that attention be given to the criminal distribution and sale of marijuana, which remains the largest source of revenue for the Mexican cartels and a cause of violence and lawlessness on both sides of the border, and "not the modest dispensaries that serve sick patients who find marijuana useful in treating pain, nausea,

Table 7.2 Fourteen States and Washington, D.C., Have Enacted Laws That Legalize Medical Marijuana

State	Year Passed	How Passed (Yes Vote)	ID Card Fee	Possession Limit	Accepts Other States' Registry ID Cards?
Alaska	1998	Ballot Measure 8 (58%)	$25/$20	1 oz. usable; 6 plants (3 mature, 3 immature)	Unknown*
California	1996	Proposition 215 (56%)	$66/$33	8 oz. usable; 18 plants (6 mature, 12 immature)*	No
Colorado	2000	Ballot Amendment 20 (54%)	$90	2 oz. usable; 6 plants (3 mature, 3 immature)	No
Hawaii	2000	Senate Bill 862 (32-18 House; 13-12 Senate)	$25	3 oz. usable; 7 plants (3 mature, 4 immature)	No
Maine	1999	Ballot Question 2 (61%)	*	2.5 oz. usable; 6 plants	Yes
Michigan	2008	Proposal 1 (63%)	$100/$25	2.5 oz. usable; 12 plants	Yes
Montana	2004	Initiative 148 (62%)	$25/$10	1 oz. usable; 6 plants	Yes

Nevada	2000	Ballot Question 9 (65%)	$150 +	1 oz. usable; 7 plants (3 mature, 4 immature)	No
New Jersey	2010	Senate Bill 119 (48-14 House; 25-13 Senate)	*	2 oz. usable	Unknown
New Mexico	2007	Senate Bill 523 (36-31 House; 32-3 Senate)	$0	6 oz. usable; 16 plants (4 mature, 12 immature)	No
Oregon	1998	Ballot Measure 67 (55%)	$100/$20	24 oz. usable; 24 plants (6 mature, 18 immature)	No
Rhode Island	2006	Senate Bill 0710 (52-10 House; 33-1 Senate)	$75/$10	2.5 oz. usable; 12 plants	Yes
Vermont	2004	Senate Bill 76 (22-7) HB 645 (82-59)	$50	2 oz. usable; 9 plants (2 mature, 7 immature)	No
Washington	1998	Initiative 692 (59%)	*	24 oz. usable; 15 plants	No

*See information source for details: http://medicalmarijuana.procon.org/view.resource.php?resourceID=000881.

Reprinted with permission of ProCon.org. "14 Legal Medical Marijuana States." June 24, 2010. http://medicalmarijuana.procon.org/viewresource.asp?resourceID=000881.

loss of appetite and other symptoms associated with serious illnesses or cancer chemotherapy" ("Good Sense" 2009).

A few days after the attorney general expressed his position on the issue, the director of the White House Office of National Drug Control Policy (ONDCP) R. Gil Kerlikowske made the following statement:

> The Department of Justice earlier this week issued guidelines for Federal prosecutors regarding laws authorizing the use of marijuana for medical purposes. . . . Advocates of marijuana legalization tried to cast the guidelines as a victory, portraying them as a step toward full legalization. Neither of these analyses is correct. Marijuana legalization, for any purpose, remains a non-starter in the Obama Administration . . .
>
> Regarding state ballot initiatives concerning "medical" marijuana, I believe that medical questions are best decided not by popular vote, but by science . . .
>
> Legalization is being sold as being a cure to ending violence in Mexico, as a cure to state budget problems, as a cure to health problems. The American public should be skeptical of anyone selling one solution as a cure for every single problem. Legalized, regulated drugs are not a panacea—pharmaceutical drugs in this country are tightly regulated and government controlled, yet we know they cause untold damage to those who abuse them.
>
> To test the idea of legalizing and taxing marijuana, we only need to look at already legal drugs—alcohol and tobacco. We know that the taxes collected on these substances pale in comparison to the social and health care costs related to their widespread use . . . Legalization would only thwart our efforts and increase the economic and social costs that result from greater drug acceptance and use. (http://www.whitehousedrugpolicy.gov/news/press09/marijuana_legalization.pdf)

INHALANTS

The category of inhalants includes volatile toxic substances, many of which are used as cleaners, adhesives, fuels, and chemical thinners. When inhaled, the substances act quickly on the central nervous system (CNS) to produce a high. Inhalant use is associated with children and young adolescents (average age 13 years), because the products are easily obtained, hidden, and used (NIDA 2010). About one million adolescents or 3.9 percent of that population use inhalants annually, and that overall number has remained the same since 2002 (SAMHSA 2009). Inhalants are the third most popular substance after marijuana and prescription drugs; however, more 12- and 13-year-olds have abused inhalants than any other category of drug (SAMHSA 2010a).

The chemicals and products involved with inhalant use make enforcement and intervention difficult. Inhalant use is a largely overlooked, major drug abuse problem. The categories of inhalants include the following:

- Volatile solvents, chemicals that vaporize at room temperature: These include fuels, such as gasoline and kerosene; substances containing the solvent toluene, such as paint and lacquer thinner and airplane glue; dry cleaning and correction fluids; felt-tip markers; and body scents, such as Axe and Lynx.
- Aerosols and propellants, such as Freon or tetrafluoroethane: These are found in whipped-cream and hair-spray canisters, spray paint, deodorants, vegetable-oil sprays for cooking, fabric-protector sprays, and computer air cleaners or air brushes, such as Dust Off. Inhaling this product has the street name "dusting." Frostbite of the lung tissue and asphyxia are real dangers of dusting.
- Volatile nitrates, such as amyl and butyl nitrate: These include locker room deodorizers and substances known as "poppers," "snappers," and "whippits." Nitrates were originally used as cardiac stimulants but graduated into use as an intoxicant and sexual enhancer. These substances are particularly associated with gay clubs.
- General anesthetics, such as nitrous oxide ("laughing gas"), chloroform, and ether: The history of inhalant use starts with the recreational ingestion of nitrous oxide and other anesthetic gases at gas frolics, parties, and brothels during the 19th century (Smith 1974).

Table 7.3 reflects the trends in past-year use of specific types of inhalants.

Inhalants are used in a variety of ways through the nose or mouth: sniffing or snorting fumes from containers; spraying aerosols directly into the nose or mouth; "bagging," which refers to sniffing or inhaling fumes from substances sprayed or deposited inside a plastic or paper bag; "huffing" from an inhalant-soaked rag stuffed in the mouth; and inhaling from balloons filled with nitrous oxide (NIDA 2010). It is difficult to generalize about the subjective effects of such a wide variety of chemicals. However, users report fast-acting and intense results, sometimes similar to that of alcohol, and the ability to stupefy and numb unwanted aspects of reality with occasional hallucinatory effects (Inaba and Cohen 2007, 306–7).

The medical consequences of inhalant abuse of particular solvents and aerosol/propellants are diverse and severely outweigh the damages from most other categories of drugs. These include asphyxiation; suffocation; convulsions and seizures; coma; choking; cardiac, respiratory, brain, lung, kidney, and bone marrow damage; risk of sudden death; and depression.

Table 7.3 Trends in Past-year Use of Specific Types of Inhalants among Past-year Initiates Aged 12 to 17, from 2002 to 2007

	2002 (%)	2003 (%)	2004 (%)	2005 (%)	2006 (%)	2007 (%)
Amyl nitrite, "poppers," locker room odorizers, or "rush"	14.0	17.0	12.6	16.4	16.5	19.3
Correction fluid, degreaser, or cleaning fluid	15.7	19.7	19.6	19.6	22.5	19.3
Gasoline or lighter fluid	26.2	23.2	25.3	26.7	27	28.1
Glue, shoe polish, or toluene	32.9	30.2	27.6	31.3	25.6	28.8
Halothane, ether, or other anesthetics	2.9	2.9	4.5	3.4	4.5	5.7
Lacquer thinner or other paint solvents	13.9	10.7	10.8	13.3	14.2	12.8
Lighter gases, such as butane or propane	9.3	9.7	9.2	8.1	7.1	9.9
Nitrous oxide or "whippits"	31.6	23.0	20.1	21.3	17.7	16.3
Spray Paints	21.4	23.3	25.4	23.9	28.1	25.1
Aerosol sprays other than spray paints	12.6	17.6	23.6	25.4	23.5	25.0

Source: SAMHSA 2009.

Inhalant Users

Most inhalant users tend to be young and use inhalants for a brief period, usually with peers in a group. Others have a short history of solitary use. The following narrative describes a young person's negative experience with inhalants as she starts to mature out and lose interest in continuing inhalant use:

> I think your right on this i too huff duster almost every other day and im begining to feel "stupid" like sometimes my words dont come outright even when im not huffing. i always tell myself i need to stop. people might say its not addicting, but i think it truly is. sometimes all i think about is getting together with some friends (that do it too) and doing it all night? ive noticed that when im on it i get real violent and rude. I would really watch for this "drug" to be around. and its right most people do not know about the duster so less likely to get caught. I kinda wish I could stay away from it its just ive done it way too much and now i cant stop. So please try to prevent it from even starting. (anonymous post on http://messageboard.inhalant.org/)

Chronic inhalant abusers, now in their late teens or early twenties, often manifest some nervous system damage, and they commonly have poor social skills and legal and employment problems (Hernandez-Avila and Pierucci-Lagha 2005). In the United States, high rates of inhalant abuse are found among incarcerated youth. For others, inhalant use is a gateway for other illicit drugs.

The WHO, to reduce the risks of inhalant abuse, has recommended control over the sale of inhalants to minors, parental education, and warning labels. Some manufacturers have begun to advertise the dangers associated with their product. For example, Falcon, the manufacturer of the cleaner Dust-Off, has warning information on the product label and on its Web site ("Inhalant Abuse" n.d.). Also, the National Conference of State Legislatures is attempting to implement uniform statutes enforcing a prohibition on sales of widely abused inhalants to minors and prohibit the deliberate ingestion of toxic vapors for the purpose of intoxication (NCSL 2010).

International Perspectives

Inhalant abuse, especially volatile solvent use is an international concern—an epidemic among young, poor street children, indigenous peoples, and poor, recent migrants to cities across five continents. American or British youths typically use inhalants to seek a cheap high and enjoy participating in rebellious peer use, but among deprived populations, inhalants are used to dull the pain of cold, hunger, sorrow, and physical abuse. Widespread use is reported in the developing and developed world (Medina-Mora and Real 2008; WHO 1998).

Several native populations of Canada suffer from catastrophic incidence of alcoholism and abuse of volatile inhalants, especially gasoline sniffing. Often, such populations are economically and culturally demoralized. One example is the Innu people of Labrador. This tribe of people was relocated from their traditional lands and hunting groups to small, isolated, and unattractive settlements offering few meaningful activities. The Innu despaired over the loss of their land, broken promises, and abusive treatment at residential mission schools. In 1999, Survival International published a report claiming that the Innu community in one location had the highest rate of suicide of any community in the world—approximately one-third of the community had attempted suicide (Samson, Wilson, and Mazower 1999). Parents were almost uniformly suffering from alcoholism; children, many of whom were abandoned, ended up inhaling gasoline from plastic bags. Severe health consequences, in addition to the high suicide rates, were rampant, including damage to eyesight, bone marrow, liver, and kidney as well as anemia. The tribal chief prevailed upon the provincial government to physically remove many of the youth for detoxification and treatment, mainly for inhalant abuse (Myers 2002).

Hallucinogenic and Dissociative Drugs (LSD and Ecstasy)

Most psychoactive drugs tend to be classified as depressants (narcotics, sedatives, alcohol, antihistamines) or stimulants (cocaine, amphetamines, caffeine). A third, very diverse category of illicit drugs—hallucinogens—includes substances that alter the way the brain processes and constructs information for the drug user. Dozens of such substances, found in cacti, mushrooms, seeds, or shrubs, have been used for thousands of years. They induce altered states of consciousness and have often been used to invoke the supernatural in ceremonial and sacred settings. The main psychedelics used in the United States have been LSD (or "acid"); psilocybin mushrooms; the peyote cactus; and mescaline, a peyote derivative mescaline. There are dozens of other hallucinogenic drugs, such as MDMA (ecstasy), and dissociative drugs, including PCP (phencyclidine or "angel dust") and ketamine (known as "Special K").

The idea that hallucinogens act to expand the consciousness and enhance the potential for personal growth emerged in the 1950s in the work of psychiatrist Humphrey Osmond, who coined the term "psychedelic," and Aldous Huxley, the author of *Brave New World*, who was an advocate for psychedelics. Under the leadership of Harvard psychologist Dr. Timothy Leary, whom President Nixon called "the most dangerous man in America," the youth counterculture of the 1960s venerated hallucinogens. Leary, in fact, had an organization called the League for Spiritual Discovery, which had the motto "Turn On, Tune In, Drop Out." Followers paired LSD use with an alternative hippie lifestyle of peace, love, and detachment from and revolt against mainstream culture, including government and medical authorities (Lee and Schlain 1985).

The 1960s is portrayed in the media and even in some drug literature as the peak period of hallucinogen use. Although the drug counterculture went out of fashion in the early 1970s, the use of hallucinogens such as LSD (and marijuana) expanded throughout the 1970s, declined during the 1980s, and had a brief comeback during the 1990s (Goode 2008, 259).

The National Institute on Drug Abuse "InfoFacts" is an information source about hallucinogens and club drugs. Two illicit drugs, LSD and ecstasy, warrant further discussion.

LSD

Lysergic acid diethylamide or LSD was discovered in 1943 by Albert Hoffman of Sandoz Pharmaceutical Company. It was derived from ergot, a fungus that may have been the basis for hallucinations experienced by residents of Salem, Massachusetts, in 1692 and the reason for witchcraft accusations there (Blumberg 2007). LSD is the most potent hallucinogen, as seen in the fact that the effective dose (ED) is measured in millionths of a gram (a microgram or "mike" in street terms). A typical dose runs from 50 to 150 micrograms, and it comes in two forms—tablets and micrograms of the drug put on blotting paper. See the figure "LSD Forms" from the U.S. Drug Enforcement Agency (2006, http://www.usdoj.gov/dea/images_lsd.html).

LSD takes effect between a half hour to an hour, peaks at about an hour and a half, after which it takes about three hours for half of the substance to leave the body. An entire LSD trip can last about 5 to 12 hours and may include many different effects. It can be exhilarating and joyous, or it can be terrifying, causing the user to feel out of control, insane, or approaching death—the infamous "bad trip" phenomenon. Chronic use of LSD can cause reoccurrences of the drug experience that are called "flashbacks" or, in clinical terminology, hallucinogen-induced persisting perceptual disorder (Inaba and Cohen 2007, 266).

LSD is not addictive; cessation of use does not produce abstinence syndrome (withdrawal). It is also not clear that LSD causes mental illness;

however, this powerful drug could worsen or trigger latent psychiatric problems. Users are typically adolescents and young adults, the ages when severe mental illnesses such as schizophrenia typically develop. Contrary to what was widely reported in the media during the 1960s and 1970s, there is little evidence that LSD causes chromosome damage and birth defects.

For years, LSD was the most commonly used hallucinogen. This is no longer the case because of its declining popularity and increasing use of psilocybin—the hallucinogenic substance found in hundreds of fungi (i.e., mushrooms)—and ecstasy (Johnston et al. 2009).

MDMA

MDMA (called "ecstasy," "XTC," "X," "E," or "Adam") is related to the amphetamine category of illicit drugs and has stimulant properties; it also has consciousness-altering or mildly hallucinogenic effects. First synthesized in 1912 by a chemist (Anton Kollisch) working for the Merck Pharmaceutical Company, MDMA appeared as a street drug in the early 1970s for relaxation and an altered state of consciousness. Over time, it has been used by psychotherapists to promote patients' communication and reduce their inhibitions, treat posttraumatic stress disorder, and help relieve anxiety related to cancer.

In the 1980s, there were parallel subcultures of MDMA users: those who championed the spiritual and interpersonal virtues of the drug, and those who merely sought recreational and euphoric drug benefits. MDMA was marketed openly in many public venues, which led the DEA to invoke emergency scheduling powers to criminalize the drug in 1985. Pro-MDMA psychiatrists bitterly opposed this measure in testimony before the DEA, but DEA attorneys responded by criticizing the therapeutic claims as scientifically unsubstantiated (Beck and Rosenbaum 2001). Despite the ban, use continued to spread to working-class and minority communities in the 1990s, and peaked in 2001, when the percentage of 12th graders who had used the drug in the previous 12 months climbed to about 9 percent from about 4 percent four years earlier (Johnston et al. 2009).

As ecstasy, MDMA (3,4-methylenedioxymethamphetamine) became a key part of the rave culture (i.e., dance parties with electronic music and light shows), and the Illicit Drug Anti-Proliferation Act of 2003 implemented harsh penalties for rave organizers, club owners, and others who allowed drugs on their premises. This action drove down its use. Ecstasy rates among high schools students rose from 1999 to 2001, dropped in 2002, and continued to decline. From 2005 to 2007 there was a rebound in use; however, in 2008, the patterns of use appear to be on the decline again—about 1 to 2 percent of high school students reported current MDMA use (Johnston et al. 2009).

Tablets usually contain 80 to 100 milligrams of MDMA and the common dosage is one or two tablets. The effects are felt in about a half hour and reach a crescendo at about an hour to an hour and a half; a total trip takes four to six hours. Ecstasy tablets are marketed with many different images (see Figure 7.1).

Users cannot be sure they are being sold pure ecstasy, and in fact, the product may contain related compounds, amphetamines, caffeine, or ephedrine. MDMA can cause a sense of euphoria and inner peace, empathy toward others, and increased energy. On the down side, after use there may be hours of restlessness, fatigue, and days of malaise. Serious complications have been reported, such as dehydration and hyperthermia related to the physical activity and dance environment (Inaba and Cohen 2007, 271).

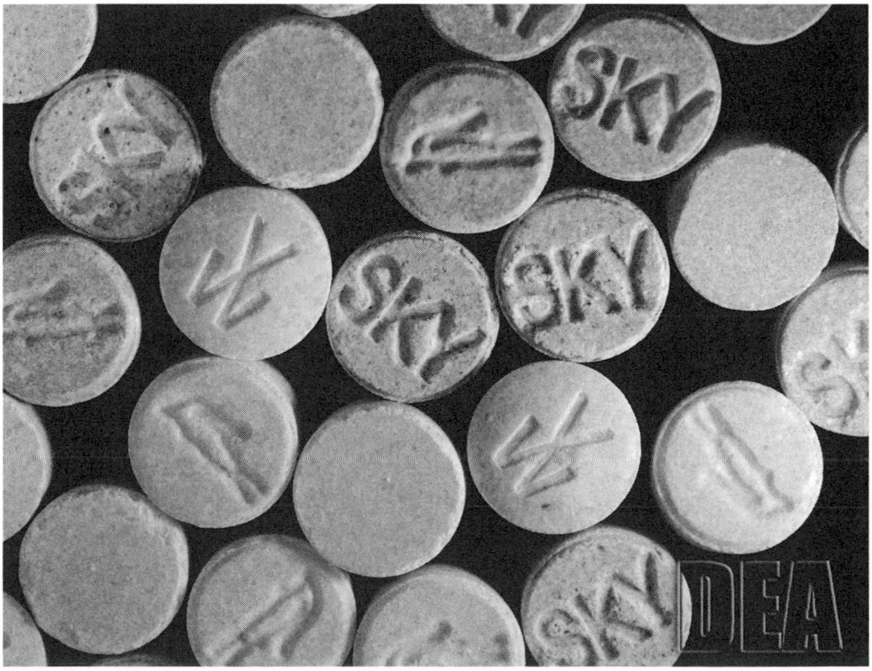

Figure 7.1 Ecstasy tablets (DEA).

Source: DEA 2003.

There has been controversy about possible damage to the brain from use of ecstasy. Research, including studies of animals, has been found to be flawed or politically inspired (Goode 2008, 269–70). For example, one study by a researcher associated with the DEA and published in *Science* stated that monkeys developed Parkinson's disease when administered MDMA (Ricaurte 2002). Upon discovery that this study was flawed, the journal retracted the article. Propagandistic presentations based on graphic visual tricks such as those purporting to show ecstasy users with holes in their brain, have been the center of ad campaigns and were featured on the *Oprah Winfrey Show*. The rampant exaggerations have led some to disavow any threat from MDMA, yet studies with scientific merit do suggest great caution in using MDMA, if not total avoidance. It is difficult to determine what a safe dose might be, and at which point the user is risking neurological damage.

Crack Cocaine

In 1983, manufacturers found a way to process cocaine to obtain a smokable and more powerful high. Regular powdered cocaine (cocaine hydrochloride or cocaine HCL) was mixed with sodium bicarbonate (baking soda) and water and then heated. This causes the alkaloid base (HCL) to separate out, leaving a pure cocaine product, albeit diluted one-third by baking soda. The product is dried into a solid form and broken into small "rocks" that weigh about 1/10 gram and burn very efficiently. The name "crack" originates from either the sound made by baking soda as it burns or the sound made by breaking the solid cake of cocaine into rocks. In rock form a single high sells for as little as five dollars, and there are none of the dangers associated with injecting drug use, such as HIV/AIDS. Thus, crack cocaine became quickly popular, especially in the inner cities of America.

The effects of crack are a rush of euphoria, exhilaration, alertness, a sense of omnipotence, increased heart rate and blood pressure, and vasoconstriction (i.e., the narrowing of blood vessels). A crack high is felt almost immediately, but lasts only 5 to 10 minutes, leaving the user irritable and depressed. As tolerance to the drug develops, users tend to gravitate toward compulsive crack use to reach that short-lived, powerful high. The effects of chronic use, coupled with the neglect of health, nutrition, and appearance that accompany the user lifestyle, produce the frightening picture of the skinny, desperate "crackhead." Lung damage, weight loss, and sexual problems are common. Seizures, strokes, and heart attacks are rare but pose a definite hazard. A terrible depression can accompany the crash at the end of a crack binge, driving the user to chase after any fragment of the drug that can be obtained at whatever cost. Those who chronically engage in crack binges may also develop a stimulant psychosis, including paranoia, hallucinations, and a feeling that insects are crawling under the skin (formication).

It is difficult for a novice health care professional to distinguish stimulant psychosis from paranoid schizophrenia, and many psychiatric inpatients were misdiagnosed as paranoid schizophrenic. In the second part of the 1980s, even the most veteran drug users were horrified at the personal and social deterioration evident among crack smokers. Stories about crack users spread through the media, including accounts of child neglect, stealing from family members, aggression, violence, and people who provided sexual favors for small amounts of the drug.

Much of the power of crack cocaine is due to the way the drug is used and affects the body:

- The lungs contain millions of tiny sacs (alveoli) with a surface area that is equal to the size of a tennis court—a huge surface for drugs to enter the body;
- There is only a microscopic distance between the alveolus and the blood. Gases and smoke have easy entrance to the bloodstream; and
- Blood from the lungs is moved directly to the brain, as opposed to the more roundabout route from the nasal membranes or even some intravenous injection sites.

As destructive as crack cocaine is, wild exaggerations developed around its use. The media was filled with references to crack babies, demonic crack mothers, the super-addictive qualities of crack, and users' propensity for violence. This amounted to a hysterical drug panic, which had consequences for the formulation of laws and sentencing guidelines.

The Crack Baby Myth

In the late 1980s, medical personnel observed that babies born to crack-using mothers had low birth weight, were irritable and impossible to sooth, and seemed neurologically impaired. These conditions were ascribed to the mothers' use of crack. Writers predicted a cost disaster for the social and education services needed to care for these babies.

A major *Washington Post* op-ed piece, "Children of Cocaine," stated, "The inner-city crack epidemic is now giving birth to the newest horror: a bio-underclass, a generation of physically damaged cocaine babies whose biological inferiority is stamped at birth...Theirs will be a life of certain suffering, of probable deviance, of permanent inferiority" (Krauthammer 1989).

Such statements, built on a preexisting image of a racial underclass, stigmatize these children and set them up for failure. Ten years later, when the generation of children born into crack was in grade school, these predictions did not hold up. Furthermore, careful studies found no difference between crack babies and other infants of the same socioeconomic group and health care status. These mothers were smoking, drinking, taking other drugs, eating junk food, and not receiving any prenatal care, all serious risk factors for infants. There has been no way to separate the crack factor from all of the other risk factors. This is not to say that crack use is safe during pregnancy. Miscarriage, premature birth, low birth weight, stress, and some developmental delays may be present (Morgan and Zimmer 1997; Frank et al. 2001).

Crack Mothers

The spread of crack cocaine was notable among women, which alarmed the public. These women, were mostly low-income, mainly African American and Latina, and often pregnant, making them the object of scorn and hostility (Humphries 1999). Admittedly, a mother addicted to a powerful stimulant will likely have serious shortcomings as a parent, but the crack mother of the late 1980s was depicted as totally abusive, immoral, and lacking in basic human qualities such as the maternal instinct. These judgments were amplified and repeated on the front pages of America's newspapers. Hospitals began secretly testing pregnant women for cocaine and reporting the results to the authorities. Tens of thousands of children were swept into foster care (Glenn 2006). By 1995, 13 states required doctors to report drug use in pregnancy or positive drug tests in newborns to law enforcement authorities. Nine states specifically defined drug use during pregnancy as child abuse or neglect and addressed this situation by means ranging from mandatory drug treatment for the mother to a criminal investigation and the possible removal of the child. By 1995, it was estimated that between 200 and 300 women had been prosecuted, often under existing child abuse and neglect statutes, and mostly for cocaine (Grieder 1995). Pregnant mothers in Michigan and South Carolina were charged with delivering drugs to a minor, even when they successfully completed drug treatment programs. The prosecution and jailing of minority crack-using mothers was way out of proportion to that for heroin-addicted mothers and white addicts. The stigma for crack mothers even percolated into drug treatment programs, where these clients already have tremendous guilt and expectations for punishment and the staff need to be especially welcoming, empathic, and nonjudgmental in order to build rapport and a treatment alliance (Myers and Salt 2007, 68–69).

Crack Sentencing

The panic over crack led the U.S. Congress to pass the Anti-Drug Abuse Acts of 1986 and 1988. Mandatory penalties for crack cocaine offenses established a vastly different structure for crack as opposed to powered cocaine. A defendant convicted of holding a mere five grams of crack cocaine (similar in volume to two sugar packets, yielding approximately 20 doses) received a mandatory five-year minimum sentence. Persons possessing powdered cocaine would have to hold 500 grams, yielding more than 2,500 doses, to receive a sentence of five years. Thus, sentencing for crack cocaine is 100 times as harsh as that for powder cocaine. The same ratio holds at higher amounts and sentences: 5,000 grams of powder and 50 grams of crack both yield a 10-year sentence. Moreover, first-time offenders possessing powder cocaine are more likely to receive probation or a short sentence rather than hard time. Crack cocaine was most prevalent in poor and minority inner-city communities, and sentencing disparities compounded the existing problem of disproportionate representation of persons of color within the criminal justice system.

By the late 1980s, the war on drugs, which was focused on crack cocaine, was a major factor for the skyrocketing prison population. Twenty-three states had a racial disparity in drug-arrest rates of more than five African Americans to one non–African American. According to a 1995 report, though African Americans accounted for only 13 percent of monthly drug users at that time, they accounted for 35 percent of all arrests for drug possession, 55 percent of all convictions for possession, and 74 percent of all prison sentences for possession (Butterfield 1995).

The Pendulum Swings

In addition to stories of crack babies and crack mothers, the drug panic of the late 1980s generated the myth that addiction occurred upon first use—even President Ronald Reagan and First Lady Nancy Reagan made such a statement (Reinarman and Levine 1997). In fact, most first-time crack users never try it again. The extent of crack use was also exaggerated; the words "crisis" and "epidemic" were commonly used, and the drug was described as being everywhere. Finally, as crack entered the marketplace, there were a huge number of small, street-level dealers who fought violent turf battles for drug sales. This violence was erroneously attributed to the pharmacological effects of the drug itself (Acker 2002).

Crack cocaine use, which spiked in the second half of the 1980s, diminished to a great extent by 1992–1993. The decrease in use was accompanied by a decrease in some of the social problems associated with crack sales, distribution, and use, such as turf wars, crack houses, and sex for crack. Many crack users had gone through treatment, died, or matured out of use by natural means. Government and medical authorities started to emphasize the removal of the stigma associated with drug use. Prisoner advocacy groups and civil rights organizations now found their voices heard when they decried the racial and socioeconomic disparities in sentencing that affected those prosecuted for crack (Sentencing Project 2010).

In 2007, the U.S. Sentencing Commission implemented new guidelines that cut the prison terms for first-time offenders possessing 5 grams or less of crack cocaine. In March 2008, over Bush administration objections, the commission's reductions were applied retroactively, allowing thousands of inmates to petition judges for shorter sentences.

State laws also have come under review. One of the most, if not the most, draconian sentencing systems was in New York State. Instituted under Governor Nelson Rockefeller in the 1970s, New York mandated huge penalties for the possession of even small amounts of illegal drugs. In March 2009, the state legislature and Governor George Pataki agreed to "Drop the Rock," as it was termed, greatly reducing penalties for first-time offenders and allowing diversion into treatment via the new drug court system.

METHAMPHETAMINE AND CRYSTAL METH

Methamphetamine (or "meth") is a powerful member of the amphetamine stimulant drug class. It was first marketed as Benzedrine in the 1930s and available without prescription for use in preventing asthma attacks, depression, and weight control. In the 1950s, a meth epidemic spread in Japan, with up to two million users injecting the drug. It is still a leading cause of drug arrests in that nation. In the late 1960s, snorted or injected amphetamine and methamphetamine became a major part of the drug culture. Aggressive, hostile, and occasionally paranoid "speed freaks" and outlaw motorcycle gangs were commonly associated with meth distribution and use throughout the 1960s and 1970s (Lee and Schlain 1985; Miller 1997, 118). Truck drivers, who had previously stayed awake on long hauls with the use of Benzedrine and other amphetamine tablets, turned to meth in the 1980s, as did gay males in the 1990s, putting them at risk for infectious disease, including—HIV/AIDS, hepatitis C, ill health, depression, loss of personal relationships, and employment problems (Kurtz 2008).

The motives for methamphetamine use vary. For example, it has been used to provide extra energy needed to work multiple jobs; subsistence through drug sales in rural, poor areas; self-medication for depression and boredom; and in urban and gay venues as a club drug (Haight et al. 2009, 29). In the mid-1980s, a more powerful, smokable form of methamphetamine known as "ice," or later as "crystal meth" or "crystal," appeared in Hawaii and then spread to California and throughout the West and Northwest during the 1990s. Epidemic use of crystal meth was predicted, but its reach throughout the country was unusually slow; it did not appear in the central or eastern United States for another decade. Associated with rural, poor, and white working-class populations, meth has had little popularity in the Northeast and among African Americans.

Meth is manufactured from the precursor chemicals ephedrine and pseudoephedrine. Ephedrine is the psychoactive ingredient found in the herb ephedra (known as ma huang in Chinese), long used to treat respiratory problems as a bronchodilator that widens the air passages of the lungs. Pseudoephedrine is a closely related synthetic substance that is used as a decongestant to reduce swelling in the sinuses. These two precursor chemicals fell under strict regulation, so meth-lab operators turned to buying over-the-counter (OTC) decongestant and cold remedies, such as Sudafed, Contac 12-Hour Caplets, among others, for what was needed to make the drug. To circumvent tighter regulation on OTC sales, meth manufacturers engaged in a practice known as "smurfing," where they drove homeless people from pharmacy to pharmacy to buy cold-remedy products. When the OTC products became regulated and the ingredients in the formulas were changed, those involved with meth labs turned to pseudoephedrine manufactured in India and China and smuggled through Mexico. The Mexican government was not able to effectively limit chemical imports from abroad until 2007, when it made major seizures of precursor chemicals. This action ultimately led to some meth shortages in the United States and the beginnings of an upswing in domestic production (NDIC 2008).

Initially, most meth was manufactured in small mom–and-pop labs with limited production. By the mid-1990s, the biker gang networks were displaced by Mexican rivals using superlabs to produce the drug. The number of reported methamphetamine laboratory seizures in the United States decreased each year from 2004 through 2008 (see Figure 7.2).

In addition to patterns of production and lab seizures, meth-treatment admissions have doubled within the decade due to such factors as the growing desperation among users, families, and communities; the availability of smokable crystal meth from Mexico; and the new availability of specialized treatment options.

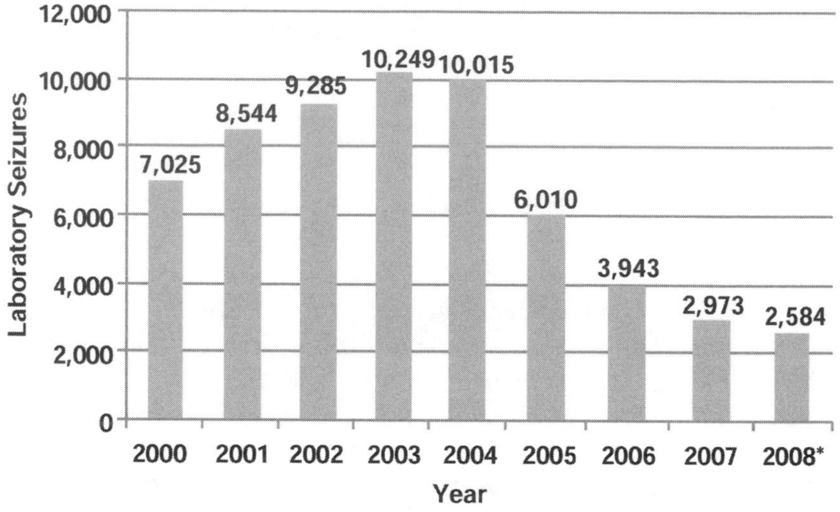

Figure 7.2 Methamphetamine laboratory seizures in the United States, 2000–2008.

*Data run November 13, 2008.

Source: National Drug Intelligence Center, National Drug Threat Assessment 2009.

The economic costs of methamphetamine abuse are comparable to those incurred by heroin. In 2007, the estimated number of past-year meth users declined from 1.9 million in 2006 to 1.3 million. However, current (i.e., past-month) users numbered 529,000, similar to the previous year. Rates of methamphetamine use among persons aged 12 years or older were the highest in the West (1.6 percent), followed by the South (0.7 percent), the Midwest (0.5 percent), and the Northeast (0.3 percent) regions of the United States (SAMHSA 2008).

The Meth Addict—Body and Mind

The physical appearance of chronic meth users reflects sickness and suffering. Meth constricts the blood vessels, causing the skin to look discolored and old, and users tend to have acne and sores that don't heal and are made worse by obsessive skin-picking. Because healthy blood flow is restricted, infection is common in users, and natural recovery from infection, even with medical intervention, is limited. The media regularly feature before-and-after pictures of meth users with blackened, rotting, and missing teeth, a condition known as "meth mouth." This phenomenon has been attributed to a lack of blood flow to the gums and to dry mouth, which prevents saliva from neutralizing acids that can eat away at teeth. Teeth grinding among "meth heads" is also common. What is omitted from many of these accounts is that the meth user likely comes from a rural area where there is very little access to dental care, dental hygiene is neglected, and where large amounts of sugary soft drinks are consumed (Daitz 2005; Richards and Brofelt 2000).

Meth users may feel alert, energized, and confident when using, but they are often anxious and irritable, lack appetite, are unable to sleep, and may engage in risky sexual behavior (Frosh et al. 1996). Multi-substance abuse is a norm with methamphetamine use; sedatives such as the Valium-like benzodiazepines, as well as alcohol, are used to soften the crash after a binge, and to smooth the anxieties and irritability that go with abuse. Heroin and methamphetamine are also used concurrently, as upper-downer "speedballs." Research has found that meth use can affect brain function, including cognition, memory, and motor skills (Volkow 2001a, 2001b).

Smokable, crystal meth is a more powerful form of the drug because it is absorbed via the alveoli in the lungs and then travels directly to the brain. This is the same principle by which crack cocaine delivers a faster and more powerful high than cocaine that is snorted or injected. Users seek a powerful euphoric high and need to use to feel normal after the crash. In communities where crystal meth is epidemic, there are serious repercussions on family and community life. One mother reported that "drugs just took over... [and] were more powerful than my love for my kids, but when you get sober, you get a heart again" (Haight et al. 2009).

Prescription Drugs

Attention and concern about the nonmedical use or abuse of prescription drugs is growing. According to the NIDA an estimated 48 million people, or 20 percent of the U.S. population aged 12 and older, have used prescription drugs for nonmedical purposes in their lifetimes. As greater access and availability have made prescription medication easier to obtain, "the total number of stimulant prescriptions in the United States has soared from around 5 million in 1991 to nearly 35 million in 2007. Prescriptions for opiates (hydrocodone and oxycodone products) have escalated from around 40 million in 1991 to nearly 180 million in 2007" (NIDA 2009).

During 2007, more than 6.9 million Americans age 12 years or older reported current (i.e., past month) nonmedical use of the three categories of prescription type drugs: (1) opioid pain relievers, such as oxycodone, morphine, and codeine; (2) CNS depressants, including tranquilizers and sedatives; and (3) stimulants (NDIC 2009). These drugs are usually prescribed for legitimate medical purposes; however, more than half (57 percent) of those reporting nonmedical use of psychotherapeutics got them "from a friend or relative for free" (SAMHSA 2008). These drugs are also obtained by improper methods such as making multiple visits to different physicians for the same health claim; visiting physicians known to run unscrupulous "prescription mills"; stealing or forging prescription pads; changing the dosage amount or number of refills indicated on a prescription; Internet sales; purchasing smuggled drugs; and/or buying stolen, forged, or fraudulently obtained prescriptions. The death of singer Michael Jackson on June 25, 2009, drew attention to these practices. According to one of his physicians "there's a plethora of doctors in Hollywood, they're drug peddlers, they're drug pushers, they just happen to be having a medical license" ("Questions Swirl" 2009).

Opioid Drugs

Opiates and opioid (narcotic analgesics or pain relievers) are the prescription drugs that are most frequently used illicitly—illicit opioid use increased fivefold between 1990 and the early 2000s. Emergency department visits for prescription opiate overdoses has skyrocketed, and the number of treatment admissions for prescription opioids as the primary drug of abuse increased 74 percent, from 114,644 in 2004 to 305,885 in 2008 (SAMHSA 2010b). According to the Centers for Disease Control and Prevention's National Center for Health Statistics, the number of deaths involving opioid analgesics was 1.93 times the number involving cocaine and 5.38 times the number involving heroin (CDC 2010).

Overdose of opioids is characterized by respiratory depression (a decrease in respiratory rate and/or volume), oscillation between apnea (i.e., the lack of breathing) and rapid breathing, cyanosis (i.e., blue coloration of the skin and mucous membranes), stupor or coma, skeletal muscle flaccidity, cold and clammy skin, slowed heartbeat, and hypotension (i.e., abnormally low blood pressure). Ultimately, circulatory collapse, respiratory arrest, cardiac arrest, and death may follow severe overdose. Fentanyl and its chemical cousin, sufentanyl, are particularly associated with fatal events as it much more powerful than heroin and morphine.

Hydrocodone and oxycodone belong to a class of narcotic medications called "opiates." These medications, often combined with acetaminophen (e.g., Tylenol) or ibuprofen (e.g., Advil), are artificial versions of the natural compounds found in opium. The brand names of these prescription painkillers include Vicodin, Percocet, Percodan, and many others. According to the National Forensic Laboratory Information System of the DEA, hydrocodone and oxycodone account for 71 percent of all narcotic pain relievers reported. The two drugs are similar, but hydrocodone is not as powerful as oxycodone. The most frequently observed adverse reactions include light-headedness, hypotension, dizziness and fainting, sedation, nausea, vomiting, sweating, weakness, dry mouth, constipation and urinary retention, muscle twitches, flushing, and skin rashes.

In the 1990s hydrocodone abuse was often considered an epidemic. "Vike" parties were described as endemic in middle-class suburbs and Hollywood circles. Yet actual use patterns are more widespread. Oxycodone was marketed by Purdue Pharma as OxyContin, a patented time-release formula designed to provide 12 hours of pain relief. Purdue thought abusers would not be able to circumvent the time-release properties of the product. However, in short order they learned to crush the microcapsules to get the benefit of the opiate high all at once. The "oxy buzz" is similar to that of other opiates: "It's a great feeling... Your body don't hurt. Nothing can bring you down... all your troubles go away... You just feel like everything is lifted off your shoulders" (user Paula, quoted in Tough 2001, 34).

Although the media forecasted a national epidemic, for the most part opiate abuse remained in Maine, Appalachia, and some rural areas of Pennsylvania and Ohio. These areas are physically remote and are characterized by high concentrations of poverty and unemployment, large numbers of chronically ill and disabled people; a local culture of prescription drug use and abuse substitutes for appropriate primary medical care and serves as a psychological and analgesic coping mechanism (Tough 2001, 34; Inciardi and Syvertsen 2008). A substance abuse counselor in rural Appalachia states:

> The factory workers I worked with in treatment, as well as the ones whom I know personally, typically use hydrocodone under the brand name of Lortab. There are several ways to obtain this particular drug here in Northwest Tennessee. Many purchase on the job site... The using employee doesn't have to go looking for the drug because the guys with the pills come to them. One of the ways is through unscrupulous doctors. At one time I could tell you the names of no less 10–20 doctors in a 100 mile radius who were known to hand out hydrocodone scripts like candy on Halloween. And [in] this 100 mile radius the states included are Tennessee, Kentucky, Missouri, Illinois and Arkansas which makes doctor-shopping easy. I was told by more than one that the prescription pads would be already completed with type and dosage and that it was just a matter of the name of the patient to be written in. Some said there were many times they didn't even see the doctor but they would get their script from the doctor's wife who worked as his nurse.
>
> I have known some personally before I ever worked in a treatment center and then worked with 100's over the past 12 years and they all tell me

> the same thing... they like the energy that the drug gives them. [It is hard to believe that they are] energized in the same sense as stimulants or is it just a matter of feeling the euphoria/sense of well being that allows them to work harder and longer? One of the most popular questions when one enters treatment is, "When will I get any energy back?" (C. Ross 2009, personal communication)

In an attempt to curb abuse of this drug, the FDA approved a slow-release version of OxyContin. The new formulation is designed to prevent the time-released pills from being "cut, broken, chewed, crushed or dissolved [by users] to release more medication" (FDA 2010).

Sedatives: The Benzodiazepines—Valium-like Drugs

Sedatives are CNS depressants. They include benzodiazepines (BZDs) or "minor tranquilizers." About 8.4 million persons (3.4 percent) aged 12 or older used sedatives for nonmedical reasons in their lifetime (SAMHSA 2008). The most common brand-name BZDs are Alprazolan, Clonazepam, and Diazepam.

Marketed in the early 1960s, BZDs became extremely popular as replacements for early, more toxic depressants such as barbiturates. About a dozen BZDs are prescribed legitimately for anxiety (the "anxiolytic" effect), sleep inducement, muscle relaxation, and to control seizure activity. At lower doses, BZDs induce calmness without undue sedation, or induce a sedation that can be counteracted with a cup of coffee. Because a person can function normally in this way, the addictive potential of BZDs is masked. At medium-range doses, BZDs induce drowsiness, slowed reaction time, impaired motor coordination, amnesia, and slurred speech. With chronic use, they may lead to depression and emotional blunting or "emotional anesthesia" (Longo and Johnson 2000). Occasionally, excitability and/or aggression may occur.

Large doses of BZDs are rarely fatal unless combined with other CNS-depressant drugs, such as opiates or alcohol. Long-term use, even in small doses, results in the development of tolerance, and ever-larger doses are required to gain the desired effect. Physical and psychological dependence also develop, and withdrawal symptoms are severe, including anxiety, irritability, insomnia, tremors, and seizures. These symptoms can persist for months, precipitating a return to usage.

BZDs are commonly used to obtain a euphoric high, and are notably associated with multiple-drug abuse. They are uncommonly the sole drug of abuse. Examples of patterns of illicit BZD use include the following: cocaine addicts use BZDs to relieve the irritability and agitation that come with cocaine binges; alcohol drinkers use BZDs to boost the high and ease withdrawal symptoms; and clients in methadone maintenance programs use them in combination with other sedative drugs to substitute for heroin, to modulate heroin withdrawal symptoms, and to boost a heroin high.

Flunitrazepam (Rohypnol) is a BZD that is illegal in the United States. Known as "roofies" or "forget me," flunitrazepam has been implicated as a date-rape drug because the tablet is dissolvable in beverages and has no evident color or taste; it also impairs short-term memory.

Stimulants

Amphetamines are powerful artificial CNS stimulants. Their effects are somewhat similar to that of cocaine but are generally more long lasting. Users find that they provide energy and confidence and reduce the need for sleep. It has been reported that more than a million prescriptions for stimulants are written each year. In 2007, an estimated 1.1 million people aged 12 years or older used stimulants nonmedically, and that included about 529,000 persons who were current users of methamphetamine (SAMSHA 2008).

Amphetamines were used by both Axis and Allied forces during World War II, by the U.S. forces during the Vietnam War in the late 1960s, and by U.S. forces in the current Afghan conflict to combat fatigue and increase alertness in soldiers and pilots. In the 1970s they were widely prescribed as appetite suppressants (anorexiants), and there was much misuse of this dietary medication because it had a euphoric effect. Subsequently, federal regulations imposed controls over this practice. Currently, amphetamines are legally prescribed for treatment of attention-deficit hyperactivity disorder (ADHD). Paradoxically, these stimulants exert a calming effect on persons with ADHD and enable them to better function in the classroom setting. Their use is highly controversial, as critics complain that ADHD is overdiagnosed and leads to overprescription of stimulants.

Amphetamine, a drug often illegally distributed and sold, has found its way to schools and to the streets for a high; to boost confidence; for its antidepressant effects, to prevent drowsiness and sleep among students, truck drivers, and construction workers; and as performance enhancers by athletes. Following the boost or high provided, users often experience a crash into exhaustion and depression, which leads the user to seek further administration of the drug. Tolerance to amphetamines also develops, leading to use of ever-higher dosages. At this point there is a risk of heart attack, stroke, and the development of a temporary amphetamine psychosis marked by aggression, suspicious, and paranoid thinking.

REFERENCES

Acker, C. 2002. *Creating the American Junkie: Addiction Research in the Classic Era of Narcotic Control.* Baltimore, Md.: Johns Hopkins University Press.

American Medical Association (AMA). 2009. Use of Cannabis for Medicinal Purposes. Available at: http://www.ama-assn.org/ama1/pub/upload/mm/443/csaph-report3-i09.pdf. Accessed September 11, 2010.

Beck, J., and R. Rosenbaum. 2001. "Emergence of Adam and Ecstasy: Distribution and Criminalization of MDMA." In *The American Drug Scene,* ed. J. Inciardi and K. McElrath. Los Angeles, Calif.: Roxbury Publishing Company.

Blumberg, J. 2007. "A Brief History of the Salem Witch Trials." Available at: http://www.smithsonianmag.com/history-archaeology/brief-salem.html. Accessed September 11, 2010.

British Home Office. 2008. "Home Office Cannabis Potency Study 2008." Available at: http://drugs.homeoffice.gov.uk/publication-search/cannabis/potency?view=Standard&pubID=553869. Accessed September 14, 2010.

Butterfield, F. 1995. "More Blacks in their 20s Have Trouble with the Law." *New York Times,* November 5, p. 18.

Canada Special Senate Committee on Illegal Drugs. 2002. "Senate Committee Recommends Legalization of Cannabis." Available at: http://www.parl.gc.ca/37/1/parlbus/commbus/senate/com-e/ille-e/press-e/04sep02-e.htm. Accessed September 10, 2010.

Centers for Disease Control (CDC). 2010. "CDC's Issue Brief: Unintentional Drug Poisoning in the United States." Available at: http://www.cdc.gov/HomeandRecreationalSafety/Poisoning/brief_full_page.htm. Accessed September 13, 2010.

Daitz, B. 2005. "Filling a Need (and a Tooth) in America's Poorest Pockets." *New York Times* (Health and Science), April 12, p. 12.

Drug Enforcement Administration (DEA). n.d. "Exposing the Myth of Smoked Medical Marijuana. Marijuana: The Facts." Available at: http://www.justice.gov/dea/ongoing/marijuana.html. Accessed February 25, 2010.

Drug Enforcement Administration (DEA). 2003. Microgram Bulletin. Available at: http://www.justice.gov/dea/programs/forensicsci/microgram/mg0103/mg0103.html. Accessed October 2, 2010.

Drug Enforcement Administration (DEA). 2010. The Controlled Substances Act: Federal Trafficking Penalties Chart. Available at: http://www.justice.gov/dea/pubs/abuse/1-csa.htm#Penalties – Marijuana. Accessed October 2, 2010.

Food and Drug Administration (FDA). 2010. "FDA Approves New Formulation for OxyContin." Available at: http://www.fda.gov/NewsEvents/Newsroom/PressAnnouncements/ucm207480.htm. Accessed April 6, 2010.

Frank, D., M. Augustyn, W. Knight, T. Pell, and B. Zuckerman. 2001. "Growth, Development, and Behavior in Early Childhood Following Prenatal Cocaine Exposure: A Systematic Review." *JAMA* 285 (12): 1613–25.

Frosh, D., S. Shoptaw, A. Huber, R. Rawson, and W. Ling 1996. "Sexual HIV Risk Among Gay and Bisexual Male Methamphetamine Abusers." *Journal of Substance Abuse Treatment* 3:483–86.

Gettman, J. 2006. "Marijuana Production in the United States." Available at: http://www.drugscience.org/Archive/bcr2/MJCropReport_2006.pdf. Accessed September 14, 2010.

Glenn, J. 2006. "The Birth of the Crack Baby and the History that 'Myths' Make." Available at: http://www.utmb.edu/addiction/Birth%20of%20the%20Crack%20Baby.pdf. Accessed September 12, 2010.

Goode, E. 2008. *Drugs in American Society,* 8th ed. New York: McGraw Hill.

"Good Sense on Medical Marijuana." 2009. *New York Times* [editorial]. Available at: http://www.nytimes.com/2009/10/21/opinion/21wed4.html. Accessed September 14, 2010.

Grieder, K. 1995. "Crackpot Ideas." *Mother Jones* (July/August). Available at: http://www.motherjones.com/politics/1995/07/crackpot-ideas. Accessed March 30, 2009.

Haight, W., J. Ostler, J. Black, and L. Kingery. 2009. *Children of Methamphetamine-Involved Families—The Case of Rural Illinois.* New York: Oxford University Press.

Hernandez-Avila, C., and A. Pierucci-Lagha. 2005. "Inhalants." In *Clinical Manual of Addiction Psychopharmacology,* ed. H. Kranzler and D. Ciraulo. Washington, D.C.: American Psychiatric Publishing.

Humphries, D. 1999. *Crack Mothers: Pregnancy, Drugs, and the Media.* Columbus: Ohio State University Press.

Inaba, D., and W. Cohen. 2007. *Uppers, Downers, and All-Arounders.* Medford, Ore.: CNS Productions.

Inciardi, J., and J. Syvertsen. 2008. "Oxycontin—Miracle Medicine or Problem Drug." In *The American Drug Scene—An Anthology,* ed. J. A. Inciardi and K. McElrath. New York: Oxford University Press.

"Inhalant Abuse: Public Awareness and Education Have Been Essential Components of Our Mission." n.d. Falcon Web site. Available at: http://www.falconsafety.com/falconsafety/inhalantabuse/default.aspx. Accessed September 11, 2010.

Johnston, L. D., P. M. O'Malley, J. G. Bachman, and J. E. Schulenberg. 2009. *Monitoring the Future: National Results on Adolescent Drug Use. Overview of Key Findings 2008.* Available at: http://monitoringthefuture.org/pubs/monographs/overview2008.pdf. Accessed June 6, 2009.

Joy J., S. Watson, and J. Benson, eds. 1999. *Marijuana and Medicine: Assessing the Science Base.* Institute of Medicine. Washington, D.C.: National Academy Press.

Krauthammer, C. 1989. "Children of Cocaine" [op-ed]. *Washington Post,* July 30, p. C7.

Kurtz, S. 2008. "Arrest Histories of High-risk Gay and Bisexual Men in Miami: Unexpected Additional Evidence for Syndemic Theory." *Journal of Psychoactive Drugs* 40 (4): 513–21.

Lee, M., and B. Schlain. 1985. *Acid Dream: The Complete Social History of LSD, the CIA, the Sixties and Beyond.* New York: Grove Press.

Longo, L., and B. Johnson. 2000. "Addiction: Part I. Benzodiazepines—Side Effects, Abuse Risk and Alternatives." *American Family Physician* 61 (7): 2121–28.

Mack, A., and J. Joy. 2000. *Marijuana as Medicine? The Science Beyond the Controversy*. Washington, D.C.: National Academy Press.

Marijuana Policy Project (MMP). 2008. "Marijuana Prohibition Facts." Available at: http://www.mpp.org/assets/pdfs/download-materials/MJ_ProhibFacts092008.pdf. Accessed June 9, 2009.

Medina-Mora, M., and T. Real. 2008. "Epidemiology of Inhalant Use." *Current Opinion in Psychiatry* 21:247–51.

Miller, M. 1997. "History and Epidemiology of Amphetamines in the United States." In *Amphetamine Misuse—International Perspectives on Current Trends*, ed. H. Klee. Amsterdam: Harwood Academic Publishers.

Morgan, J., and L. Zimmer. 1997. "The Social Pharmacology of Smokable Cocaine: Not All It's Cracked Up to Be." In *Crack in America: Demon Drugs and Social Justice,* ed. C. Reinarman and H. Levine. Berkeley: University of California Press.

Myers, P. 2002. "The Killing of the Innu." *Journal of Ethnicity in Substance Abuse* 1 (2): 1–7.

Myers, P., and N. Salt. 2007. *Becoming an Addictions Counselor: A Comprehensive Text.* Sudbury, Mass.: Jones and Bartlett.

National Commission on Marijuana and Drug Abuse. 1972. "Report: Marihuana: A Signal of Misunderstanding." Available at: http://www.druglibrary.org/schaffer/library/studies/nc/ncmenu.htm. Accessed September 10, 2010.

National Conference of State Legislatures (NCSL). 2010. "Youth Use of Inhalants and Aerosols." Available at: http://www.ncsl.org/default.aspx?tabid=16447. Accessed September 11, 2010.

National Drug Intelligence Center (NDIC). 2008. *National Methamphetamine Threat Assessment 2009.* Available at: http://www.justice.gov/ndic/pubs31/31379/meth.htm. Accessed October 2, 2010.

National Drug Intelligence Center (NDIC). 2009. *National Prescription Drug Threat Assessment 2009.* Available at: http://www.usdoj.gov/ndic/pubs33/33775/index.htm. Accessed September 14, 2010.

National Institute on Drug Administration (NIDA). 2009. "Understanding and Addressing Prescription Drug Abuse Among Adolescents." *Counselor*, June 3. Available at: http://www.counselormagazine.com/feature-articles-mainmenu-63/31-adolescents/926-understanding-and-addressing-prescription-drug-abuse-among-adolescents. Accessed June 13, 2009.

National Institute on Drug Administration (NIDA). 2010. *InfoFacts: Inhalants.* Available at: http://www.nida.nih.gov/infofacts/inhalants.html. Accessed September 11, 2010.

Office of National Drug Control Policy (ONDCP). 2009. New Report Finds Highest Levels of THC in U.S. Marijuana to Date. Available at: http://www.whitehousedrugpolicy.gov/news/press09/051409.html. Accessed September 11, 2010.

ProCon.org. 2009. "Medical Marijuana." Available at: http://medicalmarijuana.procon.org/view.resource.php?resourceID=000141. Accessed September 14, 2010.

"Questions Swirl about Jackson and Medication." 2009. CNN.com. Available at: http://edition.cnn.com/2009/SHOWBIZ/Music/06/26/michael.jackson/index.html. Accessed June 27, 2009.

Reinarman, C., and H. Levine. 1997. *Crack in America*. Berkeley: University of California Press.

Ricaurte, G., J. Yuan, G. Hatzidimitriou, B. Cord, and U. McCann. 2002. "Severe Dopaminergic Neurotoxicity in Primates after a Common Recreational Dose Regimen of MDMA ('Ecstasy')." *Science* 297 (5590): 2260–63. (See also the retraction of the article. Available at: http://www.maps.org/media/science9.5.03.html. Accessed September 14, 2010.)

Richards, J., and B. Brofeldt. 2000. "Patterns of Tooth Wear Associated with Methamphetamine Use." *Journal of Periodontology* 71 (8): 1371–74.

Runciman, R. 2000. *Drugs and the Law: Report of the Independent Inquiry into the Misuse of Drugs Act.* London: Police Foundation.

Samson, C., J. Wilson, and J. Mazower. 1999. *The Killing of the Innu: Canada's Tibet*. London, UK: Survival, Inc. Available at: http://www.survival-international.org/files/books/InnuReport.pdf. Accessed March 29, 2009.

Sentencing Project. 2010. Historic Reform: Congress Lowers Penalties for Crack Cocaine. Available at: http://www.sentencingproject.org/detail/news.cfm?news_id=966http://www.sentencingproject.org/detail/news.cfm?news_id=966. Accessed September 12, 2010.

Smith, G. 1974. *When the Cheering Stopped*. Toronto: MacLeod Publishers.

Substance Abuse and Mental Health Services Administration (SAMHSA). 2008. *Results from the 2007 National Survey on Drug Use and Health: National Findings*. Available at: http://www.oas.samhsa.gov/nsduh/2k7nsduh/2k7Results.pdf. Accessed June 15, 2009.

Substance Abuse and Mental Health Services Administration (SAMHSA). 2009. *Trends in Adolescent Inhalant Use: 2002–2007*. Available at: http://www.whitehousedrugpolicy.gov/publications/drugfact/nsduh_inhalant02-07.pdf. Accessed October 2, 2010.

Substance Abuse and Mental Health Services Administration (SAMHSA). 2010a. *New National Study Reveals 12 Year Olds More Likely to Use Potentially Deadly Inhalants than Cigarettes or Marijuana*. Available at: http://www.samhsa.gov/newsroom/advisories/1003110303.aspx. Accessed September 11, 2010.

Substance Abuse and Mental Health Services Administration (SAMHSA). 2010b. *Trends in Emergency Department Visits Involving Nonmedical Use of Narcotic Pain Relievers.* Available at: http://www.ibhinc.org/pdfs/TrendsinEmergencyDepartmentVisitsInvolvingNonmedicalUseofNarcoticPainRelievers.pdf. Accessed September 13, 2010.

Substance Abuse and Mental Health Services Administration (SAMHSA). 2010c. *Results from the 2009 National Survey on Drug Use and Health: National Findings.* Available at: http://www.drugabusestatistics.samhsa.gov/NSDUH/2k9NSDUH/2k9Results.htm. Accessed October 2, 2010

Tough, P. 2001. "The OxyContin Underground." *New York Times Magazine,* July 29, p. 31–63.

Volkow, N., L. Chang, G. Wang, J. Fowler, M. Leonido-Yee, D. Franceschi, et al. 2001a. "Association of Dopamine Transporter Reduction with Psychomotor Impairment in Methamphetamine Abusers." *American Journal of Psychiatry* 158 (3): 377–82.

Volkow, N., L. Chang, G. Wang, J. Fowler, M. Leonido-Yee, D. Franceschi, et al. 2001b. "Loss of Dopamine Transporters in Methamphetamine Abusers Recovers with Protracted Abstinence." *Journal of Neuroscience* 21 (23): 9414–18.

World Health Organization (WHO). 1998. "Volatile Solvents Abuse: A Global Overview." Available at: http://whqlibdoc.who.int/hq/1999/WHO_HSC_SAB_99.7.pdf. Accessed September 14, 2010.

Additional Readings

Angrist, B. 1994. "Amphetamine Psychosis: Clinical Variations of the Syndrome." In *Amphetamine and Its Analogs,* ed. A. Cho and D. Segal, 387–414. San Diego, Calif.: Academic Press.

Baggott, M., and J. Mendelson. 2001. "Does MDMA Cause Brain Damage?" In *Ecstasy: The Complete Guide,* ed. J. Holland. Rochester, Vt.: Inner Traditions International.

Buddy, T. 2006. "The Health Effects of Marijuana." Available at: http://alcoholism.about.com/od/pot/a/effects.htm. Accessed January 29, 2009.

Center for Substance Abuse Research (CESAR). 2008. "Nearly One-Half of Youths Who Ever Misused Prescription Pain Relievers Have Also Used Two or More Illicit Drugs." October 20. Available at: http://www.cesar.umd.edu/cesar/cesarfax/vol17/17-42.pdf. Accessed September 14, 2010.

Chavkin, W. 2001. "Cocaine and Pregnancy—Time to Look at the Evidence." *Journal of the American Medical Association* 285:1626–28.

Crider, R., and B. Rouse, eds. 1998. *Epidemiology of Inhalant Abuse: An Update.* Available at: http://www.drugabuse.gov/pdf/monographs/85.pdf. Accessed September 14, 2010.

Department of Justice. 2002. *Federal Cocaine Offenses: An Analysis of Crack and Powder Penalties.* Available at: http://www.usdoj.gov/olp/pdf/crack_powder2002.pdf. Accessed March 17, 2009.

Doweiko, H. 2009. *Concepts of Chemical Dependency.* Belmont, Calif.: Brooks-Cole.

Drug Enforcement Administration (DEA). 2005. *Drugs of Abuse*. Available at: http://www.usdoj.gov/dea/pubs/abuse/doa-p.pdf. Accessed June 27, 2009.

Drug Enforcement Administration (DEA). 2009. "Federal Trafficking Penalties." Available at: http://www.usdoj.gov/dea/agency/penalties.htm. Accessed September 20, 2010.

Dumont, R. 1988. "Abuse of Benzodiazepines—The Problems and the Solutions. A Report of a Committee of the Institute for Behavior and Health, Inc." *American Journal of Drug and Alcohol Abuse* 14 (suppl 1): 1–69.

Eiserman, J., S. Diamond, and J. Schensul. 2005. "'Rollin' on E': A Qualitative Analysis of Ecstasy Use Among Inner City Adolescents and Young Adults." In *New Drugs on the Street,* ed. M. Singer. New York: Haworth Press.

Frank, D., M. Augustyn, W. Knight, et al. 2001. "Growth, Development, and Behavior in Early Childhood Following Prenatal Cocaine Exposure: A Systematic Review." *Journal of the American Medical Association* 285:1613–25.

Harner, M. 1973. *Hallucinogens and Shamanism*. New York: Oxford University Press.

Hinds, M. de Courcy. 1990. "Instincts of Parenthood Become Part of Crack's Toll." *New York Times,* March 17, p. A1. Available at: http://www.nytimes.com/1990/03/17/us/the-instincts-of-parenthood-become-part-of-crack-s-toll.html. Accessed October 24, 2009.

Iguchi M., R. Griffiths, W. Bickel, L. Handelsman, A. Childress, and A. McLellan. 1989. "Relative Abuse Liability of Benzodiazepines in Methadone-maintained Populations in Three Cities." *NIDA Res Monogr*. 95:364–65.

Iguchi, M., L. Handelsman, W. Bickel, and R. Griffiths. 1993. "Benzodiazepine and Sedative Use/Abuse by Methadone Maintenance Clients." *Drug and Alcohol Dependence* 32 (3): 257–66.

Jacobs, M., and K. Fehr. 1987. *Drugs and Drug Abuse: A Reference Text,* 2nd ed. Toronto, Ontario: Addiction Research Foundation.

Jenkins, P. 2001. "The 'Ice Age': The Social Construction of a Drug Panic." In *The American Drug Scene—An Anthology,* 3rd ed., ed. J. Inciardi and K. McElrath. Los Angeles, Calif.: Roxbury Publishing.

Kings College London. 2009. "New Research Reveals How Cannabis Alters Brain Function." Available at: http://www.iop.kcl.ac.uk/news/?id=274. Accessed January 29, 2009.

"Marijuana." 2008. DrugWarFacts.org. Available at http://www.drugwarfacts.org/cms/?q=node/53. Accessed June 9, 2009.

Marijuana Policy Project (MPP). 2008. "Marijuana Prohibition Facts." Available at: http://www.mpp.org/assets/pdfs/download-materials/MJ_ProhibFacts092008.pdf. Accessed September 14, 2010.

Meiler, A., A. Mino, A. Chatton, and B. Broers. 2009. "Benzodiazepine Use in a Methadone Maintenance Programme: Patient Characteristics and the Physician's Dilemma." Available at: http://www.sanp.ch/pdf/2005/2005–06/2005–06–074.PDF. Accessed June 5, 2009.

Merck. 2003. "Amphetamines." *Merck Home Manual*. Available at: http://www.merck.com/mmhe/sec07/ch108/ch108g.html. Accessed June 5, 2009.

Miller, M., and N. Kozel. 1995. "Amphetamine Epidemics." In *The Encyclopedia of Drugs and Alcohol,* vol. 1, ed. J. Jaffe, 110–17. New York: Simon and Schuster.

Monitoring the Future. 2009. *U.S. High School Seniors Now as Likely to Be Smoking Cigarettes as Marijuana*. Available at: http://www.monitoringthefuture.org/data/08data/pr08t3.pdf. Accessed January 29, 2009.

National Drug Intelligence Center (NIDC). 2008. *National Drug Threat Assessment 2009*. Available at: http://www.usdoj.gov/ndic/pubs31/31379/31379p.pdf. Accessed June 6, 2009.

National Forensic Laboratory Information System (NFLIS). 2007. *Annual Report*. Available at: http://www.deadiversion.usdoj.gov/nflis/2007_annual_rpt.pdf. Accessed June 5, 2009.

National Institute on Drug Administration (NIDA). 2005a. Inhalant Abuse among Children and Adolescents: Consultation on Building an International Research Agenda, meeting summary, NIDA/Fogarty International Center, Rockville, Maryland, November 7–9, 2005. Available at: http://international.drugabuse.gov/information/PDFs/Inhalant_summary.pdf. Accessed March 29, 2009.

National Institute on Drug Administration (NIDA). 2005b. *Prescription Drugs—Abuse and Addiction*. Available at: http://www.nida.nih.gov/ResearchReports/Prescription/prescription.html. Accessed October 23, 2009.

National Institute on Drug Administration (NIDA). 2006. *Methamphetamine Abuse and Addiction*. Available at: http://www.nida.nih.gov/ResearchReports/Methamph/Methamph.html. Accessed June 6, 2009.

National Institute on Drug Administration (NIDA). 2008. "Fewer Young Adults Abuse Cocaine and Methamphetamine, National Survey Finds." Available at: http://www.nida.nih.gov/NIDA_notes/NNvol22N2/tearoff.html. Accessed September 14, 2010.

National Survey on Drug Use and Health (NSDUH). 2008a. *The NSDUH Report: Inhalant Use across the Adolescent Years*. Rockville, Md.: Substance Abuse and Mental Health Services Administration, Office of Applied Studies. Available at: http://www.oas.samhsa.gov/2k8/inhalants/inhalants.htm. Accessed March 29, 2009.

National Survey on Drug Use and Health (NSDUH). 2008b. *The NSDUH Report: Inhalant Use and Major Depressive Episode among Youths Aged 12–17*. Available at: http://www.oas.samhsa.gov/2k8/inhalantsDepress/inhalantsDepress.pdf. Accessed March 29, 2009.

National Survey on Drug Use and Health (NSDUH). 2009. *Trends in Adolescent Inhalant Use: 2002 to 2007*. Available at: http://www.oas.samhsa.gov/2k9/inhalantTrends/inhalantTrends.htm. Accessed March 29, 2009.

Paltrow, L., D. Cohen, and C. Carey. 2000. *Year 2000 Overview: Governmental Responses to Pregnant Women Who Use Alcohol or Other Drugs*. Philadelphia, Pa.: Women's Law Project, National Advocates for Pregnant Women.

Proclamation 5562. 1986. "Crack/Cocaine Awareness Month, 1986." Available at: http://www.reagan.utexas.edu/archives/speeches/1986/103186c.htm. Accessed March 30, 2009.

RAND. 2005. *The Economic Cost of Methamphetamine Use in the United States*. Available at: http://www.rand.org/pubs/monographs/MG829/. Accessed June 10, 2009.

Rasmussen, N. 2008. *On Speed: The Many Lives of Amphetamine.* New York: New York University Press.

Ratner, M., ed. 1993. *Crack Pipe as Pimp: An Ethnographic Investigation of Sex-for-crack Exchanges.* New York: Lexington Books.

Reagan, R. 1986. Address to the Nation on the Campaign Against Drug Abuse. Available at: http://www.reagan.utexas.edu/archives/speeches/1986/091486a.htm. Accessed March 21, 2009.

Reinarman, C., and H. Levine. 1997. *Crack in America, Demon Drugs and Social Justice*. Berkeley: University of California Press.

Roache, J., and R. Meisch. 1995. "Findings from Self-administration Research on the Addiction Potential of Benzodiazepines." *Psychiatric Annals* 25 (3): 153–57.

Roche, A., S. McCabe, and B. Smyth. 2008. "Illicit Methadone Use and Abuse in Young People Accessing Treatment for Opiate Dependences." *European Addiction Research* 14:219–25.

Schensul, J., S. Diamond, W. Disch, R. Bermudez, and J. Eiserman. 2005. "The Diffusion of Ecstasy through Urban Youth Networks." In *New Drugs on the Street,* ed. M. Singer. New York: Haworth Press.

Sharpe, T. 2005. *Behind the Eight Ball: Sex for Crack Exchange and Poor Black Women*. Binghamton, N.Y.: Haworth Press.

Slotkin, T. 1998. "Fetal Nicotine or Cocaine Exposure: Which One Is Worse?" *Journal of Pharmacology and Experimental Therapeutics* 285 (3): 931–45.

Stewart, O. 1987. *Peyote Religion*. Norman: University of Oklahoma Press.

The Age. 2003. "Air Force Rushes to Defend Amphetamine Use." January 18. http://www.theage.com.au/articles/2003/01/17/1042520778665.html. Accessed October 23, 2009.

Tunnell, K. 2008. "The OxyContin Epidemic and Crime Panic in Rural Kentucky." In *The American Drug Scene—An Anthology,* ed. J. Inciardi and K. McElrath. New York: Oxford University Press.

U.S. Congress. 1988. Comprehensive Anti-Drugs Act of 1988, H.R. 4842, 100th Congress. Available at: http://thomas.loc.gov/cgi-bin/bdquery/z?d100:HR04842. Accessed March 29, 2009.

U.S. Sentencing Commission (USSC). 2007. *Report to Congress: Cocaine and Federal Sentencing Policy*. Available at: http://www.ussc.gov/r_Congress/Cocaine2007.pdf. Accessed October 23, 2009.

U.S. Sentencing Commission (USSC). 2009. *Preliminary Crack Cocaine Retroactivity Data Report*. Available at: http://www.ussc.gov/USSC_Crack_Cocaine_Retroactivity_Data_Report_13_February_09.pdf. Accessed October 23, 2009.

Wilber, D. 2009. "New Sentencing Guidelines for Crack, New Challenges." *Washington Post*, January 1, p. A01. Available at: http://www.washingtonpost.com/wp-dyn/content/article/2008/12/31/AR2008123103072.html. Accessed October 24, 2009.

CHAPTER 8

Prevention and Treatment: An Overview

A major battlefront in the war against drugs is prevention and treatment. Since the 1980s, commitment to drug abuse prevention and treatment has waxed and waned under different administrations with different funding priorities responding to drug use, drug availability, and perceived national threat. For the most part, efforts have been fragmented, underfunded, and less than comprehensive for a variety of historical, political, and economic reasons, and this has created barriers to service for many people with drug problems. It has been found that every additional dollar invested in drug abuse treatment saves taxpayers $7.46 in societal costs, and domestic enforcement efforts cost 15 times as much as treatment to achieve the same reduction in societal costs (Rydell and Everingham 1994). The following description of illicit drug prevention and treatment provides a look at the issues.

PREVENTION

Prevention may be defined as those efforts that keep illicit drug problems from occurring by reducing risk factors. Whether it be a public health model or a continuum-of-care approach, the bottom line is that when illicit drugs are not used other harmful costs to society are prevented. A first line of defense is often referred to as "primary prevention." The goal of primary prevention is to increase protective factors or minimize risk factors in an environment that includes the family, school, and community to encourage abstinence from illegal drug use. The goal is to ensure that prescription and over-the-counter drugs are used only for the purposes for which they were intended and that substances that can be abused, such as gasoline, aerosols, and other inhalants, are used only for their intended purposes (CSAP 1996).

For those who have tried a drug, the goal of secondary prevention is to block harmful patterns of existing drug use and limit the progression to other, more harmful drugs. Early intervention efforts such as counseling and treatment are common in such situations. Tertiary prevention is often referred to as relapse prevention, and the goal is to address the treatment needs of chemically dependent persons.

A number of intervention strategies have demonstrated the ability to reduce or prevent drug use and drug-related crime. They include school and community-based education and prevention, drug testing and employee-assistance programs in the workplace, organized neighborhood action to drive out dealers, parenting skills classes, grassroots coalitions, and other efforts to change attitudes and promote behaviors that rule out drug use.

The provision of drug information can be an important component of a broader prevention strategy, and well-designed prevention programs can reduce drug abuse or delay onset of use. However, drug information alone does little to reduce levels of use and abuse. For example, a major graphic advertising campaign was launched in Montana in 2005 targeting methamphetamine abuse in hopes of promoting anti-methamphetamine attitudes in the state. Evaluation shows no solid evidence that the effort was effective (Erceg-Hurn 2008).

Many barriers stand in the way of prevention efforts to reduce illicit drug use. Among them are risk factors such as genetics, individual personality, age, family, community, and culture. Furthermore, it is difficult to determine whether a decline in drug use is due to specific intervention strategies or a shift in the culture. Other factors that hamper prevention efforts include the following: entrenched cultures of abuse can be quite powerful and resistant to change; communities and organizations frequently do not want to publicly acknowledge drug use in their midst; drug prevention efforts have to be repeated as new generations grow into the at-risk adolescent group; individual risk and resilience factors involve a huge therapeutic effort; and, prevention funding is inconsistent and is one of the first things to be cut from governmental budgets during hard times.

Prevention programs can succeed if planning and implementation are based on proven, scientific models of intervention (see Part III: Resources and References for evidenced-based principles for substance abuse prevention) and a well-constructed community plan that:

- Identifies the specific drugs and other child and adolescent problems in a community

- Builds on existing resources (e.g., current drug abuse prevention programs)
- Develops short-term goals related to selecting and carrying our research-based prevention programs and strategies
- Projects long-term goals so that plans and resources are available for the future
- Includes ongoing assessments of the prevention program (NIDA 2003).

Prevention efforts need to be culturally sensitive with strategies and interventions that address the family and social networks of ethnic groups, attitudes toward behavioral health and healing, religious and other community support systems, and cultural symbols such as folk and popular music (Botvin et al. 1994).

The federal government considers several prevention strategies to be evidence-based practices, which refers to methods that have been shown by objective research to promote positive change. Many of these are listed on the National Registry of Effective Programs and Practices (NREPP), a voluntary, self-nominating system in which intervention developers elect to participate. The NREPP is a searchable online registry of mental health and substance abuse interventions that have been reviewed and rated by independent reviewers. The 2010 NREPP searchable online registry includes 100 prevention interventions, including programs to strengthen communities, skills training programs, and environmental impact activities.

Treatment

Society tends to be ambivalent about the treatment of drug users. Are they evildoers who deserve punishment, sick people who should be redeemed and reclaimed, or people who should just be left to their own devices? Medical historians have noted that it is odd that drug treatment developed separately from mental health treatment in spite of an apparent link. One rcason was that physicians and psychologists did not consider drug abusers to be desirable patients. They did not comply with or pay for their treatment, they did not seem to improve, and they scared other patients out of the waiting room. However, treatment programs eventually developed out of mutual-aid movements of recovering addicts in alliance with the few professionals that stuck with them. These programs remained separate from the mainstream medical and helping professions for many decades. The *Diagnostic and Statistical Manual of Mental Disorders* (*DSM-IV-TR*), which describes behavioral health conditions requiring treatment, devotes a large section to drug abuse and drug dependency syndromes. A wide range of formal programs and mutual-aid fellowships have evolved in response to people in need of drug use treatment.

There is emerging consensus that alternatives to incarceration, such as treatment programs, are cost-effective for the criminal justice system and society. Drug treatment means fewer repeat offenders, lower medical and insurance costs, fewer accidents, and increased productivity in the workplace. Every dollar invested in treatment yields a $7 savings related to crime alone. When health care costs are factored into the equation, the savings approach $12 for every $1 invested in treatment (Belenko, Patapis, and French 2005). This new awareness has resulted in systems such as drug courts to divert drug offenders out of the criminal justice system and into treatment programs, including programs at halfway houses that combine elements of treatment and incarceration.

The Rise of Drug-Free Treatment Programs

In 1958, Charles Dederich turned his Alcoholics Anonymous group into a haven for narcotics addicts, and pioneered a confrontational, tough-love style of group encounter known as the Synanon game, so-called for the mispronounciation of "seminar" by a member. Soon, this evolved into a long-term residential program, dubbed "therapeutic communities," run by ex-addicts themselves, featuring hard work, tough love, a stratified system of status and privileges, and confrontational encounter-group meetings ranging from one- to two-hour sessions to marathon sessions lasting two days. The premise of this approach is that the addict has retreated into a psychological fortress and needs hard-hitting methods to break through their resistance and denial. Perhaps the true prototype of the therapeutic community was Daytop Village in New York, established in 1966. At Daytop, an acronym for Drug Addicts Treated on Probation, the element of love and support was added to a reentry phase of treatment to ease the client back into society. Time-extended, marathon group therapy was also pioneered there. The therapeutic community approach dominated drug treatment from the late 1960s through the 1970s. It was criticized for harsh practices, such as having members wear signs detailing their failings, and the sense that they had a cult-like, insular quality. These practices have been greatly modified at many programs since their inception. Therapeutic communities adopted reentry programs with occupational and educational training for addicts. Many staff of therapeutic communities include graduates of the program as well as professionally trained clinical staff.

Another mutual-aid movement was Narcotics Anonymous (NA), which spun off from Alcoholics Anonymous in the 1950s. Although NA remained small for its first two decades, it expanded in the 1980s. NA is a fellowship of recovering addicts following the same 12-step approach as Alcoholics Anonymous. Members believe in a spiritual awakening and reliance on a higher power as central to recovery, and they stay in touch with other members between meetings with a sponsor who plays a mentor role. NA members consider addiction to be a lifelong, chronic disease that can be held in check by taking one day at a time. NA and the therapeutic communities were on separate tracks until roughly 1990, but now many therapeutic communities encourage NA attendance on a continuing basis after graduation. Perhaps the largest alternative program is Smart Recovery, which is based on rational-emotive behavior therapy pioneered by Albert Ellis.

Core Components of Drug Treatment

For drug treatment, 13 principles suggested by NIDA form the basis of any intervention program (NIDA 2009). These principles are provided in Part III: Resources and References of this book.

Outcomes are better when treatment efforts are individualized, promote client motivation, and extend the amount of time the client is involved in the program. Drug users are not a homogeneous group, and in theory, the needs of each client should be matched to a service system characterized by rational, flexible, responsive, well-defined, short- and long-term integrated service plans developed with dependable funding resources, and ongoing monitoring and evaluation.

The core functions of comprehensive drug treatment include the following:

1. Careful screening to determine the level of severity of abuse or addiction: This determines the appropriate level of care. Also, before admission to a specific agency, screening determines whether the client is eligible and appropriate to the setting (ASAM 2001);
2. Comprehensive assessment of strengths, challenges, and readiness to change in each problem area and diagnosis;
3. Collaborative treatment planning between counselor and client to set long- and short-term goals, measurable objectives, and the means to reach them;
4. Individual, group, and family counseling;
5. Client and family education;
6. Educational and occupational services to prepare the client to reenter society as a productive citizen with a stake in a drug-free lifestyle;
7. Special attention to co-occurring psychiatric disorders: A new integrated model of treating addiction and psychiatric disorders

includes prescription of antidepressants, mood stabilizers, and antipsychotic medications and an integrated system of care; and

8. A long-term recovery maintenance plan: Because drug addiction is typically a chronic disorder characterized by occasional relapses, a short-term, one-time treatment is often not sufficient (SAMHSA/CSAT 2010).

For many, treatment is a long-term process that involves multiple interventions and attempts at abstinence. Recent research demonstrates that long-term, low-intensity recovery support is crucial. In fact, it's just as important as what is provided a patient during his stay in formal treatment (McClellan 2002; Moos 2003).

Types of Programs

Counseling and treatment of drug abuse and dependency take place in specialized programs licensed and regulated by federal and state agencies. They include the following:

- Inpatient or residential rehabilitation treatment settings,
- Intensive outpatient rehabilitation,
- Ordinary outpatient services in a clinic setting, and
- Transitional or halfway house programs after rehabilitation.

Inpatient treatment often requires a 21- to 28-day stay. This type of residential rehabilitation setting was once the gold standard of care; however, managed care constraints have resulted in the phasing out of more than half of such facilities since 1990. In addition, research shows that not everyone needs inpatient treatment. Residential care, if needed, may be offered in a medical or nonmedical facility depending on severity of the patients' problems.

A person who is physically addicted and will experience an acute abstinence or withdrawal syndrome, may need to be stabilized (that is, detoxified) in a medically managed unit if physical addiction is severe. If the addiction is relatively mild, detoxification can be managed on an outpatient basis with the support of medications to block craving and alleviate the symptoms of withdrawal. Going through detoxification does not constitute treatment, however, the repeated need for detoxification—"revolving door detox"—by a client has created the impression that drug treatment is ineffective.

Intensive outpatient rehabilitation, roughly equivalent to day treatment, is where a full range of services are provided while the patient attends the program from about 10 to 30 hours per week.

Trends in Modern Drug Treatment

Professionalization

Until the late 1970s most addiction counselors had no formal preparation and were often graduates of the same program at which they worked. Formal credentialing boards have been established in many states setting up educational standards for alcohol and drug counselors. Just as nursing and social work became professions in the 20th century, so too has addiction counseling and treatment. Some states have established a master's degree level license, and more than 400 colleges and universities have addiction counseling majors. Faculty have their own organization, INCASE, which publishes the *Journal of Teaching in the Addictions* (INCASE 2010).

Collaborative Approaches with Clients

Drug abuse treatment had, for decades, the reputation of being highly confrontational in an attempt to break through to a client supposedly in denial about her addiction. Although treatment is still more intensive and directive than general counseling and psychotherapy, it is increasingly focused on working collaboratively with clients suffering from drug dependency in a spirit of empathy and respect. It also emphasizes combating and reducing the societal and internalized stigma associated with the status of the drug user or treatment client. Although treatment still draws on the traditional therapeutic community and 12-step perspectives, there is increasing emphasis on evidence-based practices, including cognitive-behavioral therapy and motivational enhancement therapy (MET).

With MET (Miller 1995), instead of bludgeoning an abuser to accept the label of "addict" and expecting a miraculous conversion from sinner to saint, counselors recognize that even hard-core addicts want to get better on some level, and even model former addicts still have a lingering ambivalence about being clean and sober. Along with MET, the Stages of Change Model envisages addiction recovery as an upward spiral with setbacks being part of the recovery process. In this view, a mild relapse is not a catastrophe but an opportunity to learn about triggers of relapse and coping skills (Miller and Rollnick 2002; Prochaska et al. 1994).

Brief Intervention

A number of brief interventions have been found to be effective in facilitating healthy changes. Screening, Brief Intervention, and Referral to Treatment (SBIRT) is a federally sponsored initiative that stresses brief and early interventions for persons who have not become seriously chemically dependent. SBIRT is implemented in a wide variety of settings, throughout the primary health care system, emergency departments, trauma centers, schools, community institutions, and social service agencies. This is in contrast to traditional treatment, which occurs in specialized settings and addresses persons whose problems have landed them in serious trouble by the time their drug use is addressed. If screening indicates a pathological level of severity in drug use, SBIRT can refer the patient to specialized care and extensive treatment services.

Researchers from the Office of National Drug Control Policy, National Institute on Drug Abuse, and Substance Abuse and Mental Health Services Administration analyzed data from 459,599 patients who were screened for alcohol and other drug use at a variety of health care facilities, and followed up with subjects six months later to track changes in drug-use rates. The report showed that of the illicit drug users participating in SBIRT programs, 64.3 percent reported fewer arrests, 45.8 percent who were homeless said they were no longer so, and 31.2 percent reported fewer emotional problems. Also, it has been found that SBIRT programs resulted in decreases of 67.7 percent in illicit drug use rates and decreases of 38.6 percent in alcohol use rates (Madras et al. 2008).

Combination Treatment

Research indicates that a very old technique, behavioral incentives or rewards, combined with current treatment modalities, can increase perseverance in treatment, which in turn leads to completion of treatment (Budney et al. 2006). For example, a schedule of small financial rewards linked to clean urine samples or consistent attendance were combined with motivational interviewing and/or cognitive-behavioral therapy and relapse-prevention training. Separate studies indicated that this combination approach improved success rates with stimulant users, marijuana users, and patients with co-occurring psychiatric disorders (Davis 2008).

Treating Drugs with Drugs

Most people treated for dependency on opiates such as heroin or oxycodone do not receive treatment services such as those described earlier. Instead, they are enrolled in programs that offer drug substitution therapies, known as "opioid substitution therapies," which include methadone maintenance programs. Methadone hydrochloride, a synthetic narcotic, works to block opiate molecules at the specialized sites in the central nervous system. Methadone is described as a harm-reduction strategy that allows the patient to attain a legal and productive lifestyle. Methadone programs vary greatly in the degree to which they offer other services, such as counseling and education, and with which they enforce a no-tolerance policy on use of prescription sedatives, alcohol, and other drugs.

Another pharmacological intervention is suboxone, which contains a mild opiate substitute (buprenorphine) and a small amount of an opioid antagonist (naloxone). Abuse of suboxone is rare and addicts report feeling clearheaded and not sedated as is sometimes the case with methadone. Suboxone is being used to reduce illicit opioid use and help patients stay in treatment. The federal government now licenses private practice physicians to prescribe suboxone so that an addict can avoid formal treatment entirely. The drug is known colloquially as "Bupe" or "Subs."

Natural Recovery

Many former addicts did not participate in formal treatment or a recovery fellowship. Rather, they gradually diminished their use to a moderate level or became totally abstinent on their own, like those who end cigarette use without formal treatment. Many factors may contribute to what is called "natural recovery" (Granfield and Cloud 1996). For example, the addict finds the illicit drug–using lifestyle strenuous and less attractive as he ages, aspires for normal relationships and integration with society, or tires of the effects of drugs. The birth of a child or the desire for employment may also be incentives for behavior change. Many marijuana smokers, for example, complain of feeling burnt out (apathetic, emotionally blunted, depressed, and confused) as they reach their middle to late twenties. Finally, incarceration may cause an addict to rethink her life.

REFERENCES

American Society for Addiction Medicine (ASAM). 2001. *Patient Placement Criteria for the Treatment of Substance-Related Disorders,* 2nd ed., rev. Chevy Chase, Md.: ASAM.

Belenko, S., N. Patapis, and M. T. French. 2005. *Economic Benefits of Drug Treatment: A Critical Review of the Evidence for Policy Makers.* National Rural Alcohol and Drug Abuse Network. Available at: http://www.tresearch.org/resources/specials/2005Feb_EconomicBenefits.pdf. Accessed June 4, 2009.

Botvin, G. J., S. P. Schinke, J. A. Epstein, and T. Diaz. 1994. "Effectiveness of Culturally Focused and Generic Skills Training Approaches to Alcohol and Drug Abuse Prevention among Minority Youths." *Psychology of Addictive Behaviors* 8:116–27.

Budney, A., B. Moore, H. Rocha, and S. Higgins. 2006. "Clinical Trails of Abstinence-based Vouchers and Cognitive-behavioral Therapy for Cannabis Dependence." *Journal of Consulting and Clinical Psychology* 74 (2): 307–16.

Center for Substance Abuse Prevention (CSAP). 1996. *A Review of Alternative Activities and Alternative Programs in Youth-Oriented Prevention* (CSAP Technical Report No. 13). Rockville, Md.: CSAP.

Davis, D. P. 2008. "Combination Treatment Extends Marijuana Abstinence." *NIDA Notes* 21 (5): 1.

Erceg-Hurn, D. 2008. "Drugs, Money, and Graphic Ads: A Critical Review of the Montana Meth Project." *Prevention Science* 9 (4): 256–63.

Flay, B., A. Biglan, R. Boruch, et al. 2005. "Standards of Evidence: Criteria for Efficacy, Effectiveness and Dissemination." *Prevention Science* 6 (3): 151–75.

Granfield, R., and W. Cloud. 1996. "The Elephant that No-one Sees: Natural Recovery among Middle-class Addicts." *Journal of Drug Issues* 26 (1): 45–61.

International Coalition for Addiction Studies Education (INCASE). 2010. INCASE home page. Available at: http://incase-edu.net/default.aspx. Accessed September 15, 2010.

Madras, B., W. Compton, D. Avula, T. Stegbauer, J. Stein, and H. Clark. 2008. "Screening, Brief Interventions, Referral to Treatment (SBIRT) for Illicit Drug and Alcohol Use at Multiple Healthcare Sites: Comparison at Intake and 6 Months Later." *Drug and Alcohol Dependence* 99 (1): 280–95.

McClellan, A. 2002. "Have We Evaluated Addiction Treatment Correctly? Implications from a Chronic Care Perspective." *Addiction* 97:249–52.

Miller, W. 1995. "Motivational Enhancement Therapy for Drug Abusers." Available at: http://www.motivationalinterview.org/clinical/METDrugAbuse.PDF. Accessed September 15, 2010.

Miller, W., and S. Rollnick. 2002. *Motivational Interviewing: Preparing People for Change,* 2nd ed. New York: Guilford Press.

Moos, R. 2003. "Addictive Disorders in Context: Principles and Puzzles of Effective Treatment and Recovery." *Psychology of Addictive Behavior* 17 (1): 3–12.

National Institute on Drug Abuse (NIDA). 2003. *Preventing Drug Use among Children and Adolescents: A Research-Based Guide for Parents, Educators, and Community Leaders*, 2nd ed. Available at: http://www.nida.nih.gov/pdf/prevention/RedBook.pdf. Accessed September 14, 2010.

National Institute on Drug Abuse (NIDA). 2009. *Principles of Drug Addiction Treatment.* Available at: http://www.nida.nih.gov/PDF/PODAT/PODAT.pdf. Accessed September 15, 2010.

Prochaska, J., J. Norcross, and C. DiClemente. 1994. *Changing for Good.* New York: William Morrow.

Rydell, C., and S. Everingham. 1994. *Controlling Cocaine: Supply vs. Demand Programs*. Santa Monica, Calif.: Drug Policy Research Center, RAND Corporation.

Substance Abuse Mental Health Services Administration/Center for Substance Abuse Treatment (SAMHSA/CSAT). 2010. *Treatment Improvement Protocol Series.* Available at: http://www.kap.samhsa.gov/products/manuals/tips/numerical.htm. Accessed September 18, 2010.

Additional Readings

Center for Substance Abuse Prevention (CSAP). 2001. *Principles of Substance Abuse Prevention* (DHHS Publication No. [SMA]01–3507). Rockville, Md.: Center for Substance Abuse Prevention.

Greene, R., ed. 2002. *Resiliency: An Integrated Approach to Practice, Policy, and Research.* Washington, D.C.: NASW Press.

Grotberg, E. 1995. *A Guide to Promoting Resilience in Children: Strengthening the Human Spirit*. Bernard Van Leer Foundation. Available at: http://resilnet.uiuc.edu/library/grotb95b.html. Accessed March 1, 2009.

Ksir, C., C. Hart, and O. Ray. 2008. *Drugs, Society and Human Behavior*. Boston: McGraw Hill.

Myers, P. 1990. "Sources and Configurations of Institutional Denial." *Employee Assistance Quarterly* (5) 3: 43–54.

National Institute on Drug Abuse (NIDA). 1999. *Principles of Drug Addiction Treatment: A Research-Based Guide.* Available at: http://www.drugabuse.gov/PDF/PODAT/PODAT.pdf. Accessed June 11, 2009.

Newcomb, M. D., and M. Felix-Ortiz. 1992. "Multiple Protective and Risk Factors for Drug Use and Abuse: Cross-sectional and Prospective Findings." *Journal of Personality and Social Psychology* 63 (2): 280–96.

Springer, F., S. Sambrano, E. Sale, R. Kasim, and J. Hermann. 2002. *The National Cross-Site Evaluation of High-Risk Youth Programs*. Monograph Series 1. Preventing Substance Abuse: Major Findings from the National Cross-Site Evaluation of High-Risk Youth Programs. Rockville, Md.: Center for Substance Abuse Prevention.

Whitten, L. 2006. "Low-cost Incentives Improve Outcomes in Stimulant Abuse Treatment." *NIDA Notes* 21 (1). Available at: http://www.drugabuse.gov/NIDA_notes/NNvol21N1/Low.html. Accessed June 4, 2009.

PART III

Resources and References

APPENDIX A

Primary Source Documents

Illicit Drugs: Prevention and Treatment

White House Office of National Drug Control Policy

PRINCIPLES OF PREVENTION

The National Drug Control Strategy's "Performance Measures of Effectiveness" require the Office of National Drug Control Policy to "develop and implement a set of research-based principles upon which prevention programming can be based."

Evidence-Based Principles for Substance Abuse Prevention

The following 15 principles and guidelines were drawn from literature reviews and guidance supported by the federal departments of Education, Justice, and Health and Human Services as well as ONDCP. Some prevention interventions covered by these reviews have been tested in laboratory, clinical, and community settings using the most rigorous research methods. Additional interventions have been studied with techniques that meet other recognized standards. The principles and guidelines presented here are broadly supported by a growing body of research.

Address Appropriate Risk and Protective Factors for Substance Abuse in a Defined Population

1. **Define a population.** A population can be defined by age, sex, race, geography (neighbor-hood, town, or region), and institution (school or workplace).

2. **Assess levels of risk, protection, and substance abuse for that population.** Risk factors increase the risk of substance abuse, and protective factors inhibit substance abuse in the presence of risk. Risk and protective factors can be grouped in domains for research purposes (genetic, biological, social, psychological, contextual, economic, and cultural) and characterized as to their relevance to individuals, the family, peer, school, workplace, and community. Substance abuse can involve marijuana, cocaine, heroin, inhalants, methamphetamine, alcohol, and tobacco (especially among youth) as well as sequences, substitutions, and combinations of those and other psychoactive substances.
3. **Focus on all levels of risk, with special attention to those exposed to high risk and low protection.** Prevention programs and policies should focus on all levels of risk, but special attention must be given to the most important risk factors, protective factors, psychoactive substances, individuals, and groups exposed to high risk and low protection in a defined population. Population assessment can help sharpen the focus of prevention.

Use Approaches That Have Been Shown to be Effective

4. **Reduce the availability of illicit drugs, and of alcohol and tobacco for the under-aged.** Community-wide laws, policies, and programs can reduce the availability and marketing of illicit drugs. They can also reduce the availability and appeal of alcohol and tobacco to the underaged.
5. **Strengthen anti-drug-use attitudes and norms.** Strengthen environmental support for anti-drug-use attitudes by sharing accurate information about substance abuse, encouraging drug-free activities, and enforcing laws, and policies related to illicit substances.
6. **Strengthen life skills and drug refusal techniques.** Teach life skills and drug refusal skills, using interactive techniques that focus on critical thinking, communication, and social competency.
7. **Reduce risk and enhance protection in families.** Strengthen family skills by setting rules, clarifying expectations, monitoring behavior, communicating regularly, providing social support, and modeling positive behaviors.
8. **Strengthen social bonding.** Strengthen social bonding and caring relationships with people holding strong standards against substance abuse in families, schools, peer groups, mentoring programs, religious and spiritual contexts, and structured recreational activities.
9. **Ensure that interventions are appropriate for the populations being addressed.** Make sure that prevention interventions, including programs and policies, are acceptable to and appropriate for the needs and motivations of the populations and cultures being addressed.

Intervene Early at Important Stages, Transitions, and in Appropriate Settings and Domains

10. **Intervene early and at developmental stages and life transitions that predict later substance abuse.** Such developmental stages and life transitions can involve biological, psychological, or social circumstances that can increase the risk of substance abuse. Whether the stages or transitions are expected (such as puberty, adolescence, or graduation from school) or unexpected (for example the sudden death of a loved one), they should be addressed by preventive interventions as soon as possible—even before each stage or transition, whenever feasible.
11. **Reinforce interventions over time.** Repeated exposure to scientifically accurate and age-appropriate anti-drug-use messages and other interventions—especially in later developmental stages and life transitions that may increase the risk of substance abuse—can ensure that skills, norms, expectations, and behaviors learned earlier are reinforced over time.
12. **Intervene in appropriate settings and domains.** Intervene in settings and domains that most affect risk and protection for substance abuse, including homes, social services, schools, peer groups, workplaces, recreational settings, religious and spiritual settings, and communities.

Manage Programs Effectively

13. **Ensure consistency and coverage of programs and policies.** Implementation of prevention programs, policies, and messages for different parts of the community should be consistent, compatible, and appropriate.
14. **Train staff and volunteers.** To ensure that prevention programs and messages are continually delivered as intended, training should be provided regularly to staff and volunteers.
15. **Monitor and evaluate programs.** To verify that goals and objectives are being achieved program monitoring and evaluation should be a regular part of program implementation. When goals are not reached, adjustments should be made to increase effectiveness.

Source: http://www.whitehousedrugpolicy.gov/PREVENT/practice.html.

NIDA InfoFacts: Lessons from Prevention Research

The principles listed below are the result of long-term research studies on the origins of drug abuse behaviors and the common elements of effective prevention programs. These principles were developed to help prevention practitioners use the results of prevention research to address drug use among children and adolescents in communities across the country. Parents, educators, and community leaders can use these principles to help guide their thinking, planning, selection, and delivery of drug abuse prevention programs at the community level.

Prevention programs are generally designed for use in a particular setting, such as at home, at school, or within the community, but can be adapted for use in several settings. In addition, programs are also designed with the intended audience in mind: for everyone in the population, for those at greater risk, and for those already involved with drugs or other problem behaviors. Some programs can be geared for more than one audience.

Principle 1—Prevention programs should enhance protective factors and reverse or reduce risk factors (Hawkins et al. 2002).

- The risk of becoming a drug abuser involves the relationship among the number and type of risk factors (e.g., deviant attitudes and behaviors) and protective factors (e.g., parental support) (Wills et al. 1996).
- The potential impact of specific risk and protective factors changes with age. For example, risk factors within the family have greater impact on a younger child, while association with drug-abusing peers may be a more significant risk factor for an adolescent (Gerstein and Green 1993; Dishion et al. 1999).
- Early intervention with risk factors (e.g., aggressive behavior and poor self-control) often has a greater impact than later intervention by changing a child's life path (trajectory) away from problems and toward positive behaviors (Ialongo et al. 2001).
- While risk and protective factors can affect people of all groups, these factors can have a different effect depending on a person's age, gender, ethnicity, culture, and environment (Beauvais et al. 1996; Moon et al. 1999).

Principle 2—Prevention programs should address all forms of drug abuse, alone or in combination, including the underage use of legal drugs (e.g., tobacco or alcohol); the use of illegal drugs (e.g., marijuana or heroin); and the inappropriate use of legally obtained substances (e.g., inhalants), prescription medications, or over-the-counter drugs (Johnston et al. 2002).

Principle 3—Prevention programs should address the type of drug abuse problem in the local community, target modifiable risk factors, and strengthen identified protective factors (Hawkins et al. 2002).

Principle 4—Prevention programs should be tailored to address risks specific to population or audience characteristics, such as age, gender, and ethnicity, to improve program effectiveness (Oetting et al. 1997).

Principle 5—Family-based prevention programs should enhance family bonding and relationships and include parenting skills; practice in developing, discussing, and enforcing family policies on substance abuse; and training in drug education and information (Ashery et al. 1998).

Family bonding is the bedrock of the relationship between parents and children. Bonding can be strengthened through skills training on parent supportiveness of children, parent-child communication, and parental involvement (Kosterman et al. 1997).

- Parental monitoring and supervision are critical for drug abuse prevention. These skills can be enhanced with training on rule-setting; techniques for monitoring activities; praise for appropriate behavior; and moderate, consistent discipline that enforces defined family rules (Kosterman et al. 2001).
- Drug education and information for parents or caregivers reinforces what children are learning about the harmful effects of drugs and opens opportunities for family discussions about the abuse of legal and illegal substances (Bauman et al. 2001).
- Brief, family-focused interventions for the general population can positively change specific parenting behavior that can reduce later risks of drug abuse (Spoth et al. 2002b).

Principle 6—Prevention programs can be designed to intervene as early as *preschool* to address risk factors for drug abuse, such as aggressive behavior, poor social skills, and academic difficulties (Webster-Stratton 1998; Webster-Stratton et al. 2001).

Principle 7—Prevention programs for *elementary school children* should target improving academic and social-emotional learning to address risk factors for drug abuse, such as early aggression, academic failure, and school dropout. Education should focus on the following skills (Conduct Problems Prevention Research Group 2002; Ialongo et al. 2001):

- self-control;
- emotional awareness;
- communication;
- social problem-solving; and
- academic support, especially in reading.

Principle 8—Prevention programs for *middle* or *junior high* and *high school students* should increase academic and social competence with the following skills (Botvin et al. 1995; Scheier et al. 1999):

- study habits and academic support;
- communication;
- peer relationships;
- self-efficacy and assertiveness;
- drug resistance skills;
- reinforcement of anti-drug attitudes; and
- strengthening of personal commitments against drug abuse.

Principle 9—Prevention programs aimed at general populations at key transition points, such as the transition to middle school, can produce beneficial effects even among high-risk families and children. Such interventions do not single out risk populations and, therefore, reduce labeling and promote bonding to school and community (Botvin et al. 1995; Dishion et al. 2002).

Principle 10—Community prevention programs that combine two or more effective programs, such as family-based and school-based programs, can be more effective than a single program alone (Battistich et al. 1997).

Principle 11—Community prevention programs reaching populations in multiple settings—for example, schools, clubs, faith-based organizations, and the media—are most effective when they present consistent, community-wide messages in each setting (Chou et al. 1998).

Principle 12—When communities adapt programs to match their needs, community norms, or differing cultural requirements, they should retain core elements of the original research-based intervention (Spoth et al. 2002b), which include:

- Structure (how the program is organized and constructed);
- Content (the information, skills, and strategies of the program); and
- Delivery (how the program is adapted, implemented, and evaluated).

Principle 13—Prevention programs should be long-term with repeated interventions (i.e., booster programs) to reinforce the original prevention goals. Research shows that the benefits from middle school prevention programs diminish without followup programs in high school (Scheier et al. 1999).

Principle 14—Prevention programs should include teacher training on good classroom management practices, such as rewarding appropriate student behavior. Such techniques help to foster students' positive behavior, achievement, academic motivation, and school bonding (Ialongo et al. 2001).

Principle 15—Prevention programs are most effective when they employ interactive techniques, such as peer discussion groups and parent role-playing, that allow for active involvement in learning about drug abuse and reinforcing skills (Botvin et al. 1995).

Principle 16—Research-based prevention programs can be cost-effective. Similar to earlier research, recent research shows that for each dollar invested in prevention, a savings of up to $10 in treatment for alcohol or other substance abuse can be seen (Aos et al. 2001; Hawkins et al. 1999; Pentz 1998; Spoth et al. 2002a).

NIDA's prevention research program addresses all stages of child development, a mix of audiences and settings, and the delivery of effective services at the community level. The Institute focuses on risks for drug abuse and other problem behaviors that occur throughout a child's development. Prevention interventions designed and tested to address risks can help children at every step along their developmental path. Working more broadly with families, schools, and communities, scientists have found effective ways to help people gain the skills and approaches to stop problem behaviors before they occur. Research funded by NIDA and other Federal research organizations—such as the National Institute of Mental Health and the Centers for Disease Control and Prevention—shows that early intervention can prevent many adolescent risk behaviors.

References

Aos, S., Phipps, P., Barnoski, R., and Lieb, R. *The Comparative Costs and Benefits of Programs to Reduce Crime.* Vol. 4 (1–05–1201). Olympia, WA: Washington State Institute for Public Policy, May 2001.

Ashery, R.S., Robertson, E.B., and Kumpfer, K.L., eds. *Drug Abuse Prevention Through Family Interventions.* NIDA Research Monograph No. 177. Washington, DC: U.S. Government Printing Office, 1998.

Battistich, V., Solomon, D., Watson, M., and Schaps, E. Caring school communities. *Educational Psychologist* 32(3):137–151, 1997.

Bauman, K.E., Foshee, V.A., Ennett, S.T., Pemberton, M., Hicks, K.A., King, T.S., and Koch, G.G. The influence of a family program on adolescent tobacco and alcohol. *American Journal of Public Health* 91(4):604–610, 2001.

Beauvais, F., Chavez, E., Oetting, E., Deffenbacher, J., and Cornell, G. Drug use, violence, and victimization among White American, Mexican American, and American Indian dropouts, students with academic problems, and students in good academic standing. *Journal of Counseling Psychology* 43:292–299, 1996.

Botvin, G., Baker, E., Dusenbury, L., Botvin, E., and Diaz, T. Long-term follow-up results of a randomized drug-abuse prevention trial in a white middle class population. *Journal of the American Medical Association* 273:1106–1112, 1995.

Chou, C., Montgomery, S., Pentz, M., Rohrbach, L., Johnson, C., Flay, B., and Mackinnon, D. Effects of a community-based prevention program in decreasing drug use in high-risk adolescents. *American Journal of Public Health* 88:944–948, 1998.

Conduct Problems Prevention Research Group. Predictor variables associated with positive Fast Track outcomes at the end of third grade. *Journal of Abnormal Child Psychology* 30(1):37–52, 2002.

Dishion, T., McCord, J., and Poulin, F. When interventions harm: Peer groups and problem behavior. *American Psychologist* 54:755–764, 1999.

Dishion, T., Kavanagh, K., Schneiger, A.K.J., Nelson, S., and Kaufman, N. Preventing early adolescent substance use: A family centered strategy for the public middle school. *Prevention Science* 3(3):191–202, 2002.

Gerstein, D.R., and Green, L.W., eds., *Preventing Drug Abuse: What Do We Know?* Washington, DC: National Academy Press, 1993.

Hawkins, J.D., Catalano, R.F., Kosterman, R., Abbott, R., and Hill, K.G. Preventing adolescent health-risk behaviors by strengthening protection during childhood. *Archives of Pediatric and Adolescent Medicine* 153:226–234, 1999.

Hawkins, J.D., Catalano, R.F., and Arthur, M. Promoting science-based prevention in communities. *Addictive Behaviors* 90(5):1–26, 2002.

Ialongo, N., Poduska, J., Werthamer, L., and Kellam, S. The distal impact of two first-grade preventive interventions on conduct problems and disorder in early adolescence. *Journal of Emotional and Behavioral Disorders* 9:146–160, 2001.

Johnston, L.D., O'Malley, P.M., and Bachman, J.G. *Monitoring the Future National Survey Results on Drug Use, 1975–2002.* Volume 1: Secondary School Students. Bethesda, MD: National Institute on Drug Abuse, 2002.

Kosterman, R., Hawkins, J.D., Spoth, R., Haggerty, K.P., and Zhu, K. Effects of a preventive parent-training intervention on observed family interactions: Proximal outcomes from Preparing for the Drug Free Years. *Journal of Community Psychology* 25(4):337–352, 1997.

Kosterman, R., Hawkins, J.D., Haggerty, K.P., Spoth, R., and Redmond, C. Preparing for the Drug Free Years: Session-specific effects of a universal parent-training intervention with rural families. *Journal of Drug Education* 31(1):47–68, 2001.

Moon, D., Hecht, M., Jackson, K., and Spellers, R. Ethnic and gender differences and similarities in adolescent drug use and refusals of drug offers. *Substance Use and Misuse* 34(8):1059–1083, 1999.

Oetting, E., Edwards, R., Kelly, K., and Beauvais, F. Risk and protective factors for drug use among rural American youth. In: Robertson, E.B., Sloboda, Z., Boyd, G.M., Beatty, L., and Kozel, N.J., eds. *Rural Substance Abuse: State of Knowledge and Issues.* NIDA Research Monograph No. 168. Washington, DC: U.S. Government Printing Office, pp. 90–130, 1997.

Pentz, M.A. Costs, benefits, and cost-effectiveness of comprehensive drug abuse prevention. In: Bukoski, W.J., and Evans, R.I., eds. *Cost-Benefit/Cost-Effectiveness Research of Drug Abuse Prevention: Implications for Programming and Policy.* NIDA Research Monograph No. 176. Washington, DC: U.S. Government Printing Office, pp. 111–129, 1998.

Scheier, L., Botvin, G., Diaz, T., and Griffin, K. Social skills, competence, and drug refusal efficacy as predictors of adolescent alcohol use. *Journal of Drug Education* 29(3):251–278, 1999.

Spoth, R., Guyull, M., and Day, S. Universal family-focused interventions in alcohol-use disorder prevention: Cost effectiveness and cost-benefit analyses of two interventions. *Journal of Studies on Alcohol* 63:219–228, 2002a.

Spoth, R.L., Redmond, D., Trudeau, L., and Shin, C. Longitudinal substance initiation outcomes for a universal preventive intervention combining family and school programs. *Psychology of Addictive Behaviors* 16(2):129–134, 2002b.

Webster-Stratton, C. Preventing conduct problems in Head Start children: Strengthening parenting competencies. *Journal of Consulting and Clinical Psychology* 66:715–730, 1998.

Webster-Stratton, C., Reid, J., and Hammond, M. Preventing conduct problems, promoting social competence: A parent and teacher training partnership in Head Start. *Journal of Clinical Child Psychology* 30:282–302, 2001.

Wills, T., McNamara, G., Vaccaro, D., and Hirky, A. Escalated substance use: A longitudinal grouping analysis from early to middle adolescence. *Journal of Abnormal Psychology* 105:166–180, 1996.

Source: http://drugabuse.gov/infofacts/lessons.html

NIDA InfoFacts: Treatment Approaches for Drug Addiction

Drug addiction is a complex illness characterized by intense and, at times, uncontrollable drug craving, along with compulsive drug seeking and use that persist even in the face of devastating consequences. While the path to drug addiction begins with the voluntary act of taking drugs, over time a person's ability to choose not to do so becomes compromised, and seeking and consuming the drug becomes compulsive. This behavior results largely from the effects of prolonged drug exposure on brain functioning. Addiction is a brain disease that affects multiple brain circuits, including those involved in reward and motivation, learning and memory, and inhibitory control over behavior.

Because drug abuse and addiction have so many dimensions and disrupt so many aspects of an individual's life, treatment is not simple. Effective treatment programs typically incorporate many components, each directed to a particular aspect of the illness and its consequences. Addiction treatment must help the individual stop using drugs, maintain a drug-free lifestyle, and achieve productive functioning in the family, at work, and in society. Because addiction is typically a chronic disease, people cannot simply stop using drugs for a few days and be cured. Most patients require long-term or repeated episodes of care to achieve the ultimate goal of sustained abstinence and recovery of their lives.

Too often, addiction goes untreated: According to SAMHSA's National Survey on Drug Use and Health (NSDUH), 23.2 million persons (9.4 percent of the U.S. population) aged 12 or older needed treatment for an illicit drug or alcohol use problem in 2007. Of these individuals, 2.4 million (10.4 percent of those who needed treatment) received treatment at a specialty facility (i.e., hospital, drug or alcohol rehabilitation or mental health center). Thus, 20.8 million persons (8.4 percent of the population aged 12 or older) needed treatment for an illicit drug or alcohol use problem but did not receive it. These estimates are similar to those in previous years.[†]

Principles of Effective Treatment

Scientific research since the mid-1970s shows that treatment can help patients addicted to drugs stop using, avoid relapse, and successfully recover their lives. Based on this research, key principles have emerged that should form the basis of any effective treatment programs:

1. Addiction is a complex but treatable disease that affects brain function and behavior.
2. No single treatment is appropriate for everyone.
3. Treatment needs to be readily available.
4. Effective treatment attends to multiple needs of the individual, not just his or her drug abuse.
5. Remaining in treatment for an adequate period of time is critical.
6. Counseling—individual and/or group—and other behavioral therapies are the most commonly used forms of drug abuse treatment.
7. Medications are an important element of treatment for many patients, especially when combined with counseling and other behavioral therapies.
8. An individual's treatment and services plan must be assessed continually and modified as necessary to ensure that it meets his or her changing needs.
9. Many drug-addicted individuals also have other mental disorders.
10. Medically assisted detoxification is only the first stage of addiction treatment and by itself does little to change long-term drug abuse.

11. Treatment does not need to be voluntary to be effective.
12. Drug use during treatment must be monitored continuously, as lapses during treatment do occur.
13. Treatment programs should assess patients for the presence of HIV/AIDS, hepatitis B and C, tuberculosis, and other infectious diseases as well as provide targeted risk-reduction counseling to help patients modify or change behaviors that place them at risk of contracting or spreading infectious diseases.

Effective Treatment Approaches

Medication and behavioral therapy, especially when combined, are important elements of an overall therapeutic process that often begins with detoxification, followed by treatment and relapse prevention. Easing withdrawal symptoms can be important in the initiation of treatment; preventing relapse is necessary for maintaining its effects. And sometimes, as with other chronic conditions, episodes of relapse may require a return to prior treatment components. A continuum of care that includes a customized treatment regimen—addressing all aspects of an individual's life, including medical and mental health services—and followup options (e.g., community- or family-based recovery support systems) can be crucial to a person's success in achieving and maintaining a drug-free lifestyle.

Medications

Medications can be used to help with different aspects of the treatment process.

Withdrawal. Medications offer help in suppressing withdrawal symptoms during detoxification. However, medically assisted detoxification is not in itself "treatment"—it is only the first step in the treatment process. Patients who go through medically assisted withdrawal but do not receive any further treatment show drug abuse patterns similar to those who were never treated.

Treatment. Medications can be used to help reestablish normal brain function and to prevent relapse and diminish cravings. Currently, we have medications for opioids (heroin, morphine), tobacco (nicotine), and alcohol addiction and are developing others for treating stimulant (cocaine, methamphetamine) and cannabis (marijuana) addiction. Most people with severe addiction problems, however, are polydrug users (users of more than one drug) and will require treatment for all of the substances that they abuse.

- *Opioids:* Methadone, buprenorphine and, for some individuals, naltrexone are effective medications for the treatment of opiate addiction. Acting on the same targets in the brain as heroin and morphine, methadone and buprenorphine suppress withdrawal symptoms and relieve cravings. Naltrexone works by blocking the effects of heroin or other opioids at their receptor sites and should only be used in patients who have already been detoxified. Because of compliance issues, naltrexone is not as widely used as the other medications. All medications help patients disengage from drug seeking and related criminal behavior and become more receptive to behavioral treatments.

- *Tobacco:* A variety of formulations of nicotine replacement therapies now exist—including the patch, spray, gum, and lozenges—that are available over the counter. In addition, two prescription medications have been FDA-approved for tobacco addiction: bupropion and varenicline. They have different mechanisms of action in the brain, but both help prevent relapse in people trying to quit. Each of the above medications is recommended for use in combination with behavioral treatments, including group and individual therapies, as well as telephone quitlines.
- *Alcohol:* Three medications have been FDA-approved for treating alcohol dependence: naltrexone, acamprosate, and disulfiram. A fourth, topiramate, is showing encouraging results in clinical trials. Naltrexone blocks opioid receptors that are involved in the rewarding effects of drinking and in the craving for alcohol. It reduces relapse to heavy drinking and is highly effective in some but not all patients—this is likely related to genetic differences. Acamprosate is thought to reduce symptoms of protracted withdrawal, such as insomnia, anxiety, restlessness, and dysphoria (an unpleasant or uncomfortable emotional state, such as depression, anxiety, or irritability). It may be more effective in patients with severe dependence. Disulfiram interferes with the degradation of alcohol, resulting in the accumulation of acetaldehyde, which, in turn, produces a very unpleasant reaction that includes flushing, nausea, and palpitations if the patient drinks alcohol. Compliance can be a problem, but among patients who are highly motivated, disulfiram can be very effective.

Behavioral Treatments

Behavioral treatments help patients engage in the treatment process, modify their attitudes and behaviors related to drug abuse, and increase healthy life skills. These treatments can also enhance the effectiveness of medications and help people stay in treatment longer. Treatment for drug abuse and addiction can be delivered in many different settings using a variety of behavioral approaches. Outpatient behavioral treatment encompasses a wide variety of programs for patients who visit a clinic at regular intervals. Most of the programs involve individual or group drug counseling. Some programs also offer other forms of behavioral treatment such as—

- *Cognitive-behavioral therapy,* which seeks to help patients recognize, avoid, and cope with the situations in which they are most likely to abuse drugs.
- *Multidimensional family therapy,* which was developed for adolescents with drug abuse problems—as well as their families—addresses a range of influences on their drug abuse patterns and is designed to improve overall family functioning.

- *Motivational interviewing,* which capitalizes on the readiness of individuals to change their behavior and enter treatment.
- *Motivational incentives* (contingency management), which uses positive reinforcement to encourage abstinence from drugs.

Residential treatment programs can also be very effective, especially for those with more severe problems. For example, *therapeutic communities* (TCs) are highly structured programs in which patients remain at a residence, typically for 6 to 12 months. TCs differ from other treatment approaches principally in their use of the community—treatment staff and those in recovery—as a key agent of change to influence patient attitudes, perceptions, and behaviors associated with drug use. Patients in TCs may include those with relatively long histories of drug addiction, involvement in serious criminal activities, and seriously impaired social functioning. TCs are now also being designed to accommodate the needs of women who are pregnant or have children. The focus of the TC is on the resocialization of the patient to a drug-free, crime-free lifestyle.

Treatment within the Criminal Justice System

Treatment in a criminal justice setting can succeed in preventing an offender's return to criminal behavior, particularly when treatment continues as the person transitions back into the community. Studies show that treatment does not need to be voluntary to be effective.

Other Information Sources

For more detailed information on treatment approaches for drug addiction and examples of specific programs proven effective through research, view NIDA's *Principles of Drug Addiction Treatment: A Research- Based Guide* at **www.nida.nih.gov/PODAT/PODATIndex.html** (English) or **www.nida.nih.gov/PODAT/Spanish/PODATIndex.html** (Spanish).

For information about treatment for drug abusers in the criminal justice system, view NIDA's *Principles of Drug Abuse Treatment for Criminal Justice Populations: A Research-Based Guide* at **www.drugabuse.gov/PODAT_CJ.**

† Data are from the National Survey on Drug Use and Health (formerly known as the National Household Survey on Drug Abuse), which is an annual survey of Americans age 12 and older conducted by the Substance Abuse and Mental Health Services Administration. This survey is available online at **www.samhsa.gov** and from NIDA at 877–643–2644.

Source: http://www.nida.nih.gov/PDF/InfoFacts/IF_Treatment_Approaches_2009_to_NIDA_92209.pdf.

The War on Drugs and Its Impact: What Doesn't Work, What Does?

In this section, materials have been selected that reflect, in part, the range perspectives of about the war on drugs ranging from its impact on U.S. society to wasted government efforts, the controversial Drug Abuse Resistance Education program (D.A.R.E.), and an assessment of what strategies are working.

The Sentencing Project released a report in 2007 that examines the "war on drugs" and its impact on the criminal justice system and American communities. "A 25-Year Quagmire: The War on Drugs and Its Impact on American Society" assesses the strategy of combating drug abuse at the expense of investments in treatment and prevention. The following excerpt is reproduced with permission.

A 25-Year Quagmire: The War on Drugs and Its Impact on American Society

Overview

No issue has had more impact on the criminal justice system in the past three decades than national drug policy. The "war on drugs," officially declared in the early 1980s, has been a primary contributor to the enormous growth of the prison system in the United States during the last quarter-century and has affected all aspects of the criminal justice system and, consequently, American society. As a response to the problem of drug abuse, national drug policies have emphasized punishment over treatment, and in a manner that has had a disproportionate impact on low-income minority communities. After millions of people arrested and incarcerated, it is clear that the "war on drugs" has reshaped the way America responds to crime and ushered in an era of instability and mistrust in countless communities.

By the mid-1990s, the climate regarding drug policy in the United States had shifted somewhat, reflecting a growing frustration with the "lock 'em up" strategy to addressing drug abuse and growing support for the treatment model of combating drug abuse. The result was the proliferation of drug courts and other alternative sentencing strategies that sought to divert low-level drug offenders from prison into community-based treatment programs. Despite the expansion of these options over the last decade, the punitive sentencing provisions of the 1980s remain in effect across the United States, resulting in a record number of arrests, convictions, and sentences to prison for drug offenses.

Key indicators of the impact of the "war on drugs" on American communities include:

- Drug arrests have more than tripled in the last 25 years, totaling a record 1.8 million arrests in 2005;

- In 2005, 42.6% of all drug arrests were for marijuana offenses, and marijuana possession arrests accounted for 79% of the growth in drug arrests in the 1990s;
- Drug offenders in prisons and jails have increased 1,100% since 1980. Nearly a half-million (493,800) persons are in state or federal prison or local jail for a drug offense, compared to an estimated 41,100 in 1980.
- Nearly 6 in 10 persons in state prison for a drug offense have no history of violence or high-level drug selling activity;
- African Americans comprise 14% of regular drug users, but are 37% of those arrested for drug offenses and 56% of persons in state prison for drug offenses;
- African Americans serve almost as much time in federal prison for a drug offense (58.7 months) as whites do for a violent offense (61.7 months), largely due to racially disparate sentencing laws such as the 100-to-1 crack-powder cocaine disparity;
- Persons in prison with a history of regular drug use are less than half as likely to be receiving treatment as in 1991. Only 14.1% of persons in state prison in 2004 who had used drugs in the month prior to their arrest had participated in treatment compared to 36.5% in 1991. In federal prison, these proportions declined from 33.7% in 1991 to 15.2% in 2004.

The full document, M. Mauer and R. King, *A 25-Year Quagmire: The War on Drugs and Its Impact on American Society* (Washington, DC: The Sentencing Project, 2007), is available at http://www.sentencingproject.org/doc/publications/dp_25yearquagmire.pdf.

Citizens Against Government Waste released a report in 2007 that examines the government's War on Drugs"—its policies and practices. The following excerpt is reproduced with permission.

Up in Smoke: Office of National Drug Control Policy's Wasted Efforts in the War on Drugs

INTRODUCTION

Established in 1988 to oversee all aspects of America's war on drugs and to coordinate U.S. domestic and international anti-drug efforts, the White House Office of National Drug Control Policy (ONDCP) has morphed into a federal wasteland, throwing taxpayer money toward numerous high-priced drug control programs that have failed to show results. After 17 years of operation and funding, ONDCP has not achieved its objectives of reducing "illicit drug use, manufacturing, and trafficking, drug-related crime and violence, and drug-related health consequences."

Instead of curbing America's drug problem, ONDCP has wasted $4.2 billion since fiscal 1997 on media advertising, fighting state legislation, and deficient anti-drug trafficking programs. ONDCP's fiscal 2005 budget of $507 million will fund such diverse functions as local law enforcement, cracking down on medical marijuana use, drug research and treatment, and the eradication of coca crops in Latin America.

Many of ONDCP's outreach efforts focus on reducing marijuana use. In fact, since Arizona and California passed medicinal marijuana laws in November 1996, ONDCP has been intent on reducing the popularity of marijuana in the U.S. The agency created the National Youth Anti-Drug Media Campaign in 1998 just for that purpose. ONDCP also began campaigning against state ballot initiatives legalizing the use of medicinal marijuana, which is an infringement upon states' rights, a blatant misuse of tax dollars, and in contravention of ONDCP's original mission. The White House's drug office should use its resources to root out major drug operations in the U.S. instead of creating propaganda-filled news videos and flying across the country on the taxpayers' dime.

Another ONDCP program, the High Intensity Drug Trafficking Areas Program (HIDTA), has become a pork-saturated program that has been warped into a platform for cities to receive more funds for local law enforcement and small drug operations instead of being used for HIDTA's stated purpose of controlling the presence of drugs at the border. Typical of any mismanaged government-run program, members of Congress have seized upon the opportunity to ship HIDTA money to their own states and districts for political gain rather than to stop the influx of drugs. Now, states like California and Florida, which have been entitled to HIDTA monies to protect America's borders from drugs, must split funds with non-border states like Nebraska, West Virginia, and Wyoming. HIDTA cannot effectively stop drug trafficking when its resources are being diverted away from the border states. Congress has the chance to re-focus HIDTA by approving the President's fiscal 2006 budget proposal to reduce funding and consolidate the program with the Department of Justice's (DOJ) drug control programs. Rather than throwing more money at the drug problem, ONDCP should focus its resources where it will achieve the best results for taxpayers.

The full document, A. French, *Up in Smoke: Office of National Drug Control Policy's Wasted Efforts in the War on Drugs* (Washington, DC: Citizens Against Government Waste, 2005), is available at: http://www.cagw.org/assets/reports/through-the-looking-glass-reports-and-issue-briefs/2005/up_in_smoke.pdf.

Each year since 2006, presidents Bush and Obama have declared a "National D.A.R.E. Day" despite federally funded research showing the program's shortcomings. The following is the 2010 presidential proclamation.

National D.A.R.E. Day, April 8, 2010

Presidential Proclamation—National D.A.R.E. Day

A Proclamation

Every day, young Americans face pressures to engage in violent activities, drug use, and other harmful behavior. Today, we reaffirm our commitment to empowering our children to resist violence and substance abuse.

Drug dependence affects individuals from all backgrounds, and its debilitating effects often go unaddressed. Too many of our families are afflicted by addiction, and too many lives are ruined by its harmful impact. Drug abuse is not an isolated crime, and communities experience the tragic results when drug-related violence and gang activity reach our neighborhoods. It takes parents, guardians, educators, clergy, law enforcement officers, and other mentors to demonstrate that a healthy and drug-free lifestyle can build a strong foundation for future success.

Families must be vigilant in recognizing and addressing the warning signs of drug and alcohol abuse. From prescriptions and over-the-counter medications to chemical inhalants, many substances can be harmful if abused, and preventing our children from doing so is vital. I urge friends and loved ones to be role-models and to discuss the consequences of drug use with the young people in their lives.

Community-based prevention and treatment programs can provide young Americans with mentors and reinforce positive behavior. Through the Drug Abuse Resistance Education (D.A.R.E.) program, law enforcement personnel contribute their expertise to help teach America's youth to resist peer pressure, and to abstain from drugs, gangs, and violence. We all have a responsibility to join these professionals in enabling youth to choose alternatives to violence and dangerous behavior and to lead the next generation of Americans toward a brighter future.

NOW, THEREFORE, I, BARACK OBAMA, President of the United States of America, by virtue of the authority vested in me by the Constitution and the laws of the United States, do hereby proclaim April 8, 2010, as National D.A.R.E. Day. I call upon all Americans to observe this day with appropriate programs and activities.

IN WITNESS WHEREOF, I have hereunto set my hand this eighth day of April, in the year of our Lord two thousand ten, and of the Independence of the United States of America the two hundred and thirty-fourth.

BARACK OBAMA

Source: Drug Abuse Resistance Education (D.A.R.E.). 2010. National D.A.R.E. Day. Available at: http://www.dare.com/home/tertiary/default1b34.asp. Accessed October 2, 2010.

The White House Office on Drug Control Policy issued a report in 2008 titled "What Works: Effective Public Health Reponses to Drug Use." The report describes numerous government initiatives and their benefits.

What Works: Effective Public Health Responses to Drug Use

Overview

The United States has historically suffered from some of the highest rates of drug abuse in the world, and, as a result, has made unparalleled investments in demand reduction research and programming. Through hard experience, we have learned much about the nature of addiction and what works in prevention and treatment. Our policies are still evolving as we seek to incorporate the latest research findings into anti-drug programs and phase out program components that do not deliver sustained, measurable results. Now, however, ten years after the United Nations General Assembly Special Session on Drugs, it is appropriate to look back and take stock of the knowledge we have gained about what works to reduce drug abuse.

The United States National Drug Control Strategy seeks to put resources where research and experience have proven that they can have the greatest effect in reducing the demand for drugs in America. The results achieved over the last six years are particularly clear and instructive. Current use of any illicit drug among young people in America has declined by 24 percent since 2001. Youth marijuana use has fallen by 25 percent, MDMA (Ecstasy) by 54 percent, LSD by 60 percent, amphetamines by 32 percent, methamphetamine by 64 percent, and steroids by 33 percent. Use of alcohol and tobacco among American youth has also declined significantly (by 15 percent and 33 percent, respectively) suggesting a broad shift in youth attitudes and behavior. These results illustrate what can be achieved through the implementation of a balanced strategy that focuses on research-proven approaches.

It is our hope that the significant investments made by the United States in the area of drug research and program evaluation can serve to benefit nations around the world that are confronting drug abuse problems of their own. In an effort to make this hope a reality, we have produced this publication for the international community as a guide to the demand reduction efforts that have produced results in the United States.

We know that many nations now face the kinds of drug abuse problems that the United States has faced for decades. Perhaps it is inevitable. Over time, improvements in communications, travel, and technology have made our world smaller and have dramatically improved the quality of life for people around the globe. However, this interconnectedness has also led to the globalization of problems that at one time may have been considered local, national, or regional. Drug abuse has truly become such a global problem, impacting many societies in ways that they have not seen before. Although the international community has made great strides in strengthening its collective fight against drug abuse, there is still much that we can learn from each other.

In this booklet we highlight several of the cost-effective, research-tested demand reduction initiatives that have proven successful in the United States and could be helpful to countries around the world in addressing their own drug abuse challenges. The following pages will focus on such proven initiatives as

- Launching a comprehensive youth anti-drug media campaign
- Building successful community coalitions
- Employing drug testing in the workplace and at schools

- Screening and intervening to interrupt the cycle of drug abuse
- Providing quality drug treatment services at low cost
- Establishing drug treatment courts

In addition to sharing our experiences with these programs, we would like to invite readers to explore the wealth of information available from U.S. research institutions such as the National Institute on Drug Abuse (NIDA). Much of this information has been summarized and organized at the Office of National Drug Control Policy (ONDCP) web site, www.whitehousedrugpolicy.gov. Even more information, including links to thousands of peer-reviewed journal articles, is available at the National Institute for Drug Abuse (NIDA) web site, www.nida.gov.

NIDA plays a critical role in helping to shape effective, evidence-based prevention and treatment strategies. NIDA researchers have been conducting groundbreaking research into how drugs of abuse affect a user's brain and behavior, including the roles played by genetics, environment, age, gender, and other factors. By improving our understanding of addiction, NIDA-supported research can help to determine which measures are most effective in preventing drug abuse. In the area of treatment, NIDA-supported research is offering new hope through research into medications that can reduce an addict's urge to use, or that can chemically prevent a drug from entering a user's brain.

Of course, as is highlighted in the section of this document on drug free community coalitions, drug problems vary not only by nation, but also by region, city, and town. Nonetheless, we believe at least some of the work conducted in the United States will prove useful in the design and implementation of effective programs in other countries. We hope that the knowledge gained from drug research conducted by institutions like NIDA can help nations make the tough decisions about where to invest limited resources to confront the difficult problem of drug abuse.

The full document can be found at ONDCP, *What Works: Effective Public Health Responses to Drug Use* (Washington, DC: ONDCP, 2008), available at: http://www.ncjrs.gov/ondcppubs/publications/pdf/whatworks.pdf.

APPENDIX B

Commonly Abused Drugs: Categories and Street Terms

SUBSTANCES

Categories and Names	Commercial and Street Names
Cannabinoids	
Hashish	*Street*: boom, chronic, gangster, hash, hash oil, hemp
Marijuana	*Street*: blunt, dope, ganja, herb, joint, Mary Jane, pot, reefer, sinsemilla, weed
Depressants	
Barbiturates	*Commercial*: Amytal, Nembutal, Seconal, phenobarbital *Street*: barbs, reds, red birds, phennies, tooies, yellows, yellow jackets
Benzodiazepines (other than flunitrazepam)	*Commercial*: lorazepam (Ativan), triazolam (Halcion), chlordiazepoxide (Librium), diazepam (Valium), alprazolam (Xanax), clonazepam (Klonopin), clorazepate (Tranxene), oxazepam (Serax) *Street*: candy, downers, sleeping pills, tranks, benzos
Flunitrazepam	*Commercial*: Rohypnol *Street*: forget-me-pill, Mexican Valium, R2, Roche, roofies, roofinol, rope, rophies
GHB	*Commercial*: gamma-hydroxybutyrate

	Street: G, Georgia home boy, grievous bodily harm, liquid ecstasy
Methaqualone	*Commercial*: Quaalude, Sopor, Parest *Street*: ludes, mandrex, quad, quay, disco biscuits

Dissociative Anesthetics

Ketamine	*Commercial*: Ketalar SV *Street*: cat Valiums, K, Special K, vitamin K
PCP and analogs	*Commercial*: phencyclidine *Street*: angel dust, boat, hog, love boat, peace pill

Hallucinogens

LSD	*Commercial*: lysergic acid diethylamide *Street*: acid, blotter, boomers, cubes, microdot, yellow sunshines
Mescaline	*Street*: buttons, cactus, mesc, peyote
Psilocybin	*Street*: magic mushroom, purple passion

Opioids and Morphine Derivatives

Codeine	*Commercial*: Empirin with codeine, Fiorinal with codeine, Robitussin A-C, Tylenol with codeine *Street*: Captain Cody, Cody, schoolboy (with glutethimide—a hypnotic sedative), hits, doors & fours, loads, pancakes and syrup
Fentanyl	*Commercial*: Actiq, Duragesic, Sublimaze *Street*: Apache, China girl, China white, dance fever, friend, goodfella, jackpot, murder, 8, TNT, Tango and Cash
Heroin	*Commercial*: diacetylmorphine *Street*: brown sugar, dope, H, horse, junk, skag, skunk, smack, white horse
Morphine	*Commercial*: Roxanol, Duramorph *Street*: M, Miss Emma, monkey, white stuff
Opium	*Commercial*: laudanum, paregoric *Street*: big O, black stuff, block, gum, hop
Meperidine	*Commercial*: Demerol *Street*: Demmies

Hydromorphone	*Commercial*: Dilaudid *Street*: D, dillies, dust, Footballs, juice, smack
Oxycodone	*Commercial*: Oxycontin; oxycodone with acetaminophen: Percocet, Oxycet, Roxicet, Tylox *Street*: OC, Oxy, Ox, Oxycotton, hillbilly heroin
Hydrocodone (with acetaminophen)	*Commercial:* Vicodin, Lortab, Lorcet, Hydrocet *Street:* Vikes
Methadone	*Commercial:* Symoron, Dolophine, Amidone, Methadose *Street*: Dollies, Fizzies, Meth

Stimulants

Amphetamine	*Commercial*: Biphetamine, Dexedrine *Street*: bennies, black beauties, crosses, hearts, LA turnaround, speed, truck drivers, uppers
Cocaine	*Commercial*: cocaine hydrochloride *Street*: blow, bump, C, candy, Charlie, coke, crack, flake, rock, snow, toot
MDMA	*Commercial:* methylenedioxymeth-amphetamine *Street*: 007s, 69s, Adam, B-bombs, Batmans, Bean, Dex, Diamonds, Lover's speed, Smurfs, Snackies
Methamphetamine	*Commercial*: Desoxyn *Street*: chalk, crank, crystal, fire, glass, go, fast, ice, meth, speed
Methylphenidate	*Commercial*: Ritalin *Street*: JIF, MPH, R-ball, Skippy, the smart drug, vitamin R
Nicotine	*Street*: bidis, chew, cigars, cigarettes, smokeless tobacco, snuff, spit tobacco

Other Compounds

Anabolic steroids	*Commercial*: Anadrol, Oxandrin, Durabolin, Depo-Testosterone, Equipoise; *Street*: roids, juice

Inhalants	*Commercial*: Solvents (paint thinners, gasoline, glues), gases (butane, propane, aerosol propellants, nitrous oxide), nitrites (isoamyl, isobutyl, cyclohexyl) *Street*: laughing gas, poppers, snappers, whippets

ADDITIONAL READINGS

Friedman, D., and S. Rusche. 1999. Glossary. In *False Messengers: How Addictive Drugs Change the Brain*, Amsterdam, The Netherlands: Harwood Academic Publishers, Reprinted in the Addiction Studies Program Web site. Available at: http://www.addictionstudies.org/glossary.html. Accessed June 19, 2009.

Office of National Drug Control Policy. "Street Terms." Available at: http://www.whitehousedrugpolicy.gov/streetterms. Accessed June 19, 2009.

United Nations International Drug Control Programme. 2000. *Demand Reduction: A Glossary of Terms*. Available at: http://www.unodc.org/pdf/report_2000-11-30_1.pdf. Accessed June 19, 2009.

US NO Drugs. Handling Addiction and Restoring Lives. Available at: http://www.usnodrugs.com/glossary.htm. Accessed September 16, 2010.

APPENDIX C

Basic Psychopharmacology of Illicit Drugs

Like individual personality, family, peer relations, and community, basic chemistry and biology of the human body are factors that are related to illicit drug use. The following brief description provides an overview of the role of the chemistry and biology of the body play a role in illicit drug use.

Drugs enter the body in the following ways (i.e., routes of administration):

- Smoking is the most rapid and effective method of getting high from a drug. The surface area of the alveoli (tiny sacs) of the lungs is huge, so smoked drugs have a large area to enter the bloodstream. In addition, the route from the lungs to the brain is most direct. Crack cocaine, for example, is the most powerful form of that drug because it is smoked.
- Injecting is the next most effective route of administration and this is subdivided into following methods (listed in terms of effectiveness):
  - Injection directly into the bloodstream
  - Intramuscular injection into muscle tissue; and
  - Subcutaneous injection just under the surface of the skin, which is called "skin popping"
- Snorting drugs (e.g., a line of cocaine) into the nose where it is absorbed.
- Oral use of a liquid or pill, which is slow and the least effective route of drug taking.
- Transdermal patches send a slow, small, measured amount of a drug, usually a painkiller, into the body. Addicts often use any way of obtaining drugs, so transdermal patches, including those that contain fentanyl (a powerful synthetic narcotic), have been stolen from pharmacies as an opiate substitute.

Drugs and the Nervous System

Illicit drugs discussed in this book affect communication and body control, which are linked to the body's nervous systems:

- The central nervous system, which consists of the brain and spinal cord, is where information is gathered and processed. Mind, mood, perception, learning, and memory are involved.
- The somatic nervous system carries sensory information to the central nervous system and sends messages to the muscles to activate movement.
- The autonomic nervous system regulates involuntary body functions such as heartbeat and respiration (Hart, Ksir, and Ray 2009, 85–86).

Drug Interactions

Drug interactions occur when different drugs are taken together. Two similar drugs taken together may have an additive effect. For example, if one ingests two tablets of diazepam (Valium) and two tablets of clonazepam (Klonopin), it will have the effect of taking four tablets of either drug.

On the other hand, when two dissimilar drugs are taken together, one drug may offset the effect of another; this is called an *antagonistic* effect. A sedative, for example, can bring down a person high on cocaine. Illicit drugs may hinder the effects of important medications, such as those taken for blood thinning or clotting, diabetes, and high blood pressure. Some drugs taken together may have more than an additive effect; this is referred to as a multiplying or *synergistic* effect. For example, barbiturate sedatives taken with even modest amounts of alcohol accounted for many overdoses.

Adaptation to the Effects of Drugs: Key Terms

Tolerance occurs when the drugs being used no longer have the desired effect, which necessitates an increase in use. *Physiological tolerance* occurs, for example, when the liver produces more enzymes to accelerate the metabolic oxidation of a drug to eliminate it from the body more rapidly, or where the neurons become more insensitive to the effects of a drug. *Behavioral tolerance* occurs when the user learns to compensate for the effect of a drug.

Cross-tolerance means that if a person is tolerant to one drug, that person is also tolerant to other drugs in that class. For example, a heroin user will be tolerant to other narcotics, and a cocaine user will be tolerant to amphetamines.

Therapeutic index, or margin of safety, is the difference between the effective dose (ED), that is, the dose required to achieve the desired effect, and the lethal dose (LD), or the amount that will kill the user. Some drugs, such as benzodiazepines (i.e., minor tranquilizers) with trade names such as Valium, Xanax, Serax, Ativan, Klonopin, Librium and Tranxene, are very commonly prescribed as anti-anxiety drugs or anxiolytics. There is a wide difference between what will sedate and what will kill a person. With the development of physiological tolerance, both the ED and the LD may go up; a long-time user, for example, may speak clearly under the influence of an amount that would kill a novice user of sedatives. However, the margin of safety may narrow, as with the case of barbiturates, where the amount needed to get high (the ED) goes up over time, but the lethal dose (LD) does not go up proportionally. Another consideration is when a person takes an ED of a sedative drug, say, to induce sleep, but has not yet felt the effects and then because of drug-added confusion loses track of the amount ingested. This may lead to an LD.

Drug dependence refers to physiological and psychological dependence. Physiological dependence is when a person feels adverse effects (*abstinence syndrome, withdrawal syndrome*) upon cessation of use. In a withdrawal reaction, there is often the reverse of the drug effects. Thus, a person detoxing from a depressant may be irritable and have insomnia. A person who discontinues the use of stimulants may experience a crash accompanied by severe depression and fatigue. In addition, opiate withdrawal resembles an intestinal influenza with vomiting, diarrhea, cramps, chills, and aches. Withdrawal from benzodiazepines (Valium, Halcion, Klonopin, Xanax, Ativan) may involve insomnia, agitation, muscle twitching, and seizures.

Drug abuse versus drug dependence is distinguished by many sets of criteria. In general, however, drug abuse refers to use that continues despite known negative consequences to the user and/or his family or associates. Drug dependence or addiction adds the dimension of compulsive use, inability to abstain, and loss of control. Official psychiatric criteria for diagnosing drug abuse, drug dependence, intoxication and withdrawal are presented in the *Diagnostic and Statistic Manual of Mental Disorders IV- TR* (APA 2000).

Cross dependence refers to substituting drugs within a class of drugs to forestall withdrawal syndromes. For example, heroin addicts may use the synthetic opiate methadone for treatment purposes; this is also known as opioid substitution therapy.

Drug elimination from the body occurs when the drug is broken down in the body or metabolized at measurable rates. The pharmacological term for the period of time necessary for the body to eliminate half of the drug ingested is called the "half-life." Thus, THC (tetrahydrocannabinol), the active ingredient in marijuana, has a half-life of about 20 hours, which means that 20 hours after smoking pot, half of the drug remains in the body. In another 20 hours, one-fourth of the drug remains in the body. If a person smokes pot every two days, the body will still contain residues from the previous usage. Drugs are broken down into breakdown products or metabolites. For example, marijuana metabolites linger in fatty tissues for weeks and thus are detectable by drug tests for a lengthy period, as opposed to, say, LSD, which leaves the body within hours.

Drugs and brain-based psychiatric disorders, including organically based mental illnesses such as schizophrenia and manic-depression, are not caused by illicit drug use. Drug intoxication and withdrawal syndromes may mimic or resemble mental illness, especially when they generate hallucinations and perceptual distortions; when paranoid thinking occurs, as with the stimulant psychoses; and when bizarre behavior is present, as with angel dust/PCP intoxication. Chronic use of depressants and, to a lesser extent marijuana, contributes to the development and worsening of depression.

Dual diagnosis is a determination when a drug user also suffers from a mental illness (referred to as a dual or co-occurring disorder). Drug use can worsen the symptoms of mental illness, or precipitate a flare-up of symptoms where there has been relative stability. One of the paradoxes of co-occurring disorders is that persons with psychiatric disorders may be able, to some extent, to self-medicate with the use of illicit drugs.

From abuse to addiction refers to the fact that drug abuse has vicious cycles that often lead to drug dependence or addiction. These cycles include physiological and behavioral tolerance, as outlined earlier; impaired motor skills; and memory, judgment, and problem-solving abilities that lead to negative health and social consequences, including a higher level of psychological pain, depression, sense of helplessness, and lower self-esteem. There may also be a tendency among users, as well as members of their families and peer group, to deny, avoid, minimize, or explain away the worsening abuse and rescuing behavior attempts that include the need to confront unpleasant realities.

References

American Psychiatric Association (APA). 2000. *Diagnostic and Statistical Manual of Mental Disorders,* 4th ed., text rev. Washington, D.C.: APA.

Hart, C., C. Ksir, and O, Ray. 2009. *Drugs, Society, and Human Behavior,* 13th ed. New York: McGraw-Hill.

Additional Readings

Brunton, L., ed. 2006. *Goodman and Gilman's The Pharmacological Basis of Therapeutics,* 11th ed. New York: McGraw-Hill.

Degenhardt, L., W. Hall, M. Lynskey, and C. Coffee. 2004. "The Association Between Cannabis Use and Depression: A Review of the Evidence." In *Marijuana and Madness*, ed. D. J. Castle and R. Murray. Cambridge: Cambridge University Press.

Inaba, D., and W. Cohen. 2007. *Uppers, Downers, and All-Arounders,* 6th ed. Medford, Ore.: CNS Productions.

Mignon, S., M. Faiia, P. Myers, and E. Rubington. 2009. *Substance Use and Misuse—Exploring Alcohol and Drug Issues.* Boulder, Colo.: Lynn Reiner Publishers.

Myers, P., and N. Salt. 2009. *Becoming an Addictions Counselor: A Comprehensive Text,* 2nd ed. Sudbury, Mass.: Jones and Bartlett.

APPENDIX D

Chronology

The following chronology includes significant events, decisions, policies, and agreements that relate to illicit drug use.

1872 California passes the first anti-opium (i.e., laudanum—an opium preparation) law in the United States.

1881 California passes a law targeting commercial places, such as opium dens frequented by Chinese immigrants, making it a misdemeanor to maintain a place where opium was sold, given away, or smoked.

1906 Congress passes the first Pure Food and Drug Act, which requires that medicines containing opiates and certain other drugs must say so on their labels. Later amendments to the act also require that the quantity of each drug be stated on the label, and that the drugs meet official standards of identity and purity (Brecher et al. 1972).

1909 First international meeting on drugs is held in Shanghai, China, to discuss opium. The United States supports of a total ban on opium. Britain, fearing the loss of its valuable trade, opposes the plan. Thirteen nations attend but no international treaty comes out of the conference.

The United States Congress passes the Act to Prohibit the Importation and Smoking of Opium and the Opium Exclusion Act making it criminal to buy and sell opium for nonmedicinal purposes.

1912 The Hague Convention for the Suppression of Opium and Other Drugs requires the production, sale, and use of opium, heroin, morphine, and cocaine to be limited to medical and other legitimate purposes. Both the United States and Italy want cannabis included in the convention, but they are unsuccessful.

1913 Congress passes the Harrison Act, which regulates and taxes the production, importation, and distribution of opiates. This law is considered to a cornerstone of U.S. drug policy and is a key step in the criminalization of drugs and the war on drugs.

1916 The case *United States v. Coca Cola Company of Atlanta* is brought before the Supreme Court. The suit alleges that Coca-Cola is adulterated and misbranded. The court rules in favor of the company declaring that Coca-Cola is the distinctive name of the product under which it had been known and sold for more than 20 years as an article of food and is not in violation of the Food and Drugs Act provisions.

1919 The U.S. Supreme Court upholds the Harrison Act (in *United States v. Doremus*) as a valid exercise of the taxing power.

1922 The Narcotics Drug Import and Export Act (also known as the Jones-Miller Act) is passed to eliminate the use of narcotics except for legitimate medicinal use. The legislation also establishes the Federal Narcotics Control Board (in the Treasury Department).

1925 In *Linder v. United States*, the U.S. Supreme Court rules that narcotics agents have no legal right to interfere in the medical prescription of narcotics—even if the prescription is solely intended to maintain a narcotics addict on her drug of choice. This is a major legal setback to the supporters of the narcotics laws who want to stop narcotics maintenance as a moral issue. In response, the narcotics agents get around the ruling by indicting 15,000 people in the following years (by their own records) but do not bring any of them to trial simply because they know they will lose in court. The indictments, however, are sufficient to instill enough fear to permanently stop all medical attempts at narcotics maintenance in the United States (Schaffer Library on Drug Policy 2010a).

1926 In *United States v. Daugherty* the defendant is convicted of three separate offenses of sale of cocaine and receives three consecutive five-year sentences. The court rules that it is legal to treat all three offenses as separate offenses for sentencing.

1929 The Porter Narcotic Farm Act authorizes the construction of two hospitals for drug addicts and the creation of a Public Health Service (PHS) Narcotics Division. The first hospital is built in Lexington, Kentucky, in 1935, and the second facility opens in Fort Worth, Texas, in 1938. These facilities were prisons modified to provide medical and psychiatric services.

1930 The Federal Bureau of Narcotics is created in the Treasury Department under a Commissioner of Narcotics. The bureau is an enforcement structure under the direction of Commissioner

Harry Anslinger—a former railroad investigator married to the niece of Andrew W. Mellon, the secretary of the U.S. Treasury, who appointed him to his 32-year post as commissioner. The Federal Bureau of Narcotics is one of the predecessors to the current Drug Enforcement Agency (DEA).

1932 Congress passes the Uniform State Narcotic Act to encourage states to control marijuana use and research its connection to crime. By 1937 every state prohibits marijuana use, an approach the Federal Bureau of Narcotics endorses as an alternative to federal laws.

1936 *Reefer Madness*, originally titled *Tell Your Children*, is a film about the tragic events that follow when pushers lure high school students to try "marihuana"; a killing, a suicide, a rape, and a descent into madness all ensue. Some sources have claimed that the film was financed by Harry Anslinger's Federal Bureau of Narcotics, by anti-hemp interests such as DuPont, or by William Randolph Hearst. The movie is still a cult classic.

1937 The Marihuana Tax Act imposes special taxes on persons engaged in marijuana-related activities. Passage of the act makes nonmedical use of marijuana illegal. Only the birdseed industry, which argues that hemp seeds give birds' feathers a particularly shiny gloss, is exempted from the act. The Marihuana Tax Act effectively bans recreational and medicinal use of cannabis in the United States. The act also authorizes the secretary of the Treasury (then Andrew Mellon) to grant the commissioner (then Harry Anslinger) and agents of the Treasury Department's Bureau of Narcotics absolute administrative regulatory and police powers in the enforcement of the law.

"Marihuana is an addictive drug which produces in its users insanity, criminality, and death." The American Medical Association goes on record stating "There is no evidence... that the medicinal use of [cannabis and its preparations and derivatives] has caused or is causing cannabis addiction" (Woodward 1937).

1942 The Opium Poppy Act passes prohibiting the cultivation of the opium poppy except under license in the United States.

1944 The New York Academy of Medicine publishes the LaGuardia Report, which examines the social, medicinal, and legal aspects of marijuana. The report concludes, among other things, that marijuana does not lead to addiction.

1946 The Narcotics Act gives the Federal Bureau of Narcotics authority over synthetic narcotics that could be demonstrated as being addictive.

1951 The Boggs Act is the first major drug legislation passed since the 1937 Marihuana Tax Act. In response to an apparent increase in illicit drug use among minority populations in many northern cities, the act calls for mandatory minimum federal sentences for drug offenders.

1956 The Narcotics Manufacturing Act is put into effect imposing harsher penalties than before. Narcotics agents are given permission to make arrests without warrants, and drug users, drug addicts, and drug offenders are made to register at the border when entering or leaving the country.

1960 The Narcotics Manufacturing Act tightens controls and restrictions over legally manufactured narcotic drugs.

The Single Convention on Narcotic Drugs, an international treaty, creates a legal framework for combating trafficking in narcotic drugs and drug abuse, including the early identification, treatment, education, after care, rehabilitation, and social reintegration of the persons involved. The convention does not specify what those measures should be, leaving this to the individual signatories to define. The convention proposes outlawing cannabis use and cannabis cultivation worldwide and eradicating cannabis smoking within 30 years (by 1991). The U.S. representative to the convention is Harry Anslinger.

President Kennedy appoints the Prettyman Commission, or Advisory Commission on Narcotic and Drug Abuse. Among its recommendations are to decrease the use of minimum mandatory sentences, increase appropriations for research, and transfer the Federal Bureau of Narcotics to the Department of Health, Education, and Welfare.

1961 Soon after his inauguration, President Kennedy initiates action to have Harry Anslinger retire or be removed from his leadership role with the Federal Bureau of Narcotics.

1962 California has a law against being an addict is challenged when Larry Robinson is convicted based on the testimony of two policemen who say he had needle marks and admitted addiction. Robinson and his defense attorneys say the conviction is unconstitutional. In *Robinson v. California*, the U.S. Supreme Court agrees, stating that one's "status" does not constitute a crime.

1963 The Community Mental Health Centers Act promotes the establishment of community-based treatment centers. It is one of the first legislative acts to focus attention on drug treatment.

1965 The Drug Abuse Control Amendment puts control of non-narcotic drugs, such as amphetamines, barbiturates, and hallucinogenic substances, under the federal government.

1966 The Narcotic Addict Rehabilitation Act specifies narcotics addiction as a mental illness and initiates a federally sponsored national program for long-term treatment and rehabilitation of narcotic addicts.

1968 The Alcoholic and Narcotic Addict Rehabilitation Amendments authorize grants for the construction of narcotic treatment facilities in the states and for specialized training programs and materials for prevention and treatment of narcotic addiction.

1969 Dr. Timothy Leary is charged with possession of marijuana. He argues that the Marihuana Tax Act is unconstitutional on the grounds that it requires self-incrimination in order to comply with the law. The U.S. Supreme Court agrees with Leary in *Leary v. United States*, and it overturns the Marihuana Tax Act on constitutional grounds.

1970 The Comprehensive Drug Abuse and Prevention and Control Act expands the national drug abuse program by extending the services of federally funded community treatment centers to non-narcotic drug abusers and addicts.

President Richard Nixon creates the National Commission on Marijuana and Drug Abuse to review national drug policy.

Congress passes the Racketeer-Influenced and Corrupt Organizations Act and the Continuing Criminal Enterprise statute. Both laws call for the forfeiture of ill-gotten gain and the removal of the rights of drug traffickers to any personal assets or property (e.g., real estate, cash, automobiles, and jewelry) obtained by or used in a criminal business or activity.

1972 The 1970 National Commission on Marijuana and Drug Abuse report *Marijuana: A Signal of Misunderstanding* is released. The report recommends the elimination of criminal penalties for possession of small amounts of marijuana. Noting that half the nation's young people admit using marijuana, the commission argues that relying on the criminal justice system to reduce drug use is neither practical nor effective. Ten states adopt decriminalization laws, and Alaska makes marijuana possession legal.

1973 On July 1 the Drug Enforcement Administration (DEA) is created. The DEA's mission is to enforce the controlled substances laws and regulations of the United States and bring to the criminal and civil justice system of the United States, or any other competent jurisdiction, those organizations and principal members of organizations, involved in the growing, manufacture, or distribution of controlled substances appearing in or destined for illicit traffic in the United States; and to recommend and support non-enforcement programs aimed at reducing the availability of illicit controlled substances on the domestic and international markets (DEA 2010).

1974 The National Institute on Drug Abuse is established as part of the Alcohol, Drug Abuse, and Mental Health Administration. It serves as the lead federal agency for conducting basic, clinical, and epidemiological research to improve the understanding, treatment, and prevention of drug abuse and addiction and the health consequences of these behaviors.

Testifying before the Select Committee on Narcotics Abuse and Control, officials in the Carter administration state that the federal government does not have a specific treatment program for marijuana, and in fact, the administrator of the Federal Alcohol, Drug Abuse and Mental Health Agency says, "There is no treatment required for the use of marijuana as such" (U.S. House of Representatives, Select Committee on Narcotics Abuse and Control 1978a, 8). The officials also state that "we have talked about the propriety of decriminalizing the possession of small amounts of marijuana for personal use, under Federal statute only. This would, in effect, merely codify what is already occurring, since Federal law enforcement efforts should not be directed at people who possess small amounts of any drug, particularly marijuana" (U.S. House of Representatives, Select Committee on Narcotics Abuse and Control 1978b, 8). Finally, they affirm that the federal position under the Carter administration is that the move toward decriminalization is a state-by-state choice and should not be mandated by the federal government.

1980 The National Organization for the Reform of Marijuana Laws (NORML) asks the U.S. Supreme Court to overturn the Controlled Substances Act prohibition on private possession of marijuana. The court declares in *NORML v. Bell* that it is its responsibility "to construe and enforce the Constitution and laws of the land as they are and not to legislate social policy on the basis of . . . personal inclinations or other nonlegal considerations" (Schaffer Library on Drug Policy 2010b).

1984 The Comprehensive Crime Control Act broadens criminal and civil asset forfeiture laws and increases federal criminal sanctions for drug offenses.

1986 President Reagan signs the Anti-Drug Abuse Act, which mandates sentences for drug-related crimes. In conjunction with the Comprehensive Crime Control Act of 1984, the new law raises federal penalties for marijuana possession and dealing, basing the penalties on the amount of the drug involved. Possession of 100 marijuana plants receives the same penalty as possession of 100 grams of heroin. The act, considered to be racially biased, establishes mandatory 6- and 10-year prison terms for drug dealing, as well as the 100-to-1 ratio of crack to cocaine in which possession of 5 grams of crack cocaine triggers the same prison sentence as possession of 500 grams of powder cocaine. A life sentence now requires the sale of just 3.3 pounds of crack. A later amendment to this act establishes a three strikes and you're out policy, requiring life sentences for repeat drug offenders and providing for the death penalty for drug kingpins.

1988 The Anti-Drug Abuse Amendment Act raises federal penalties for marijuana possession, cultivation, and trafficking. Sentences are to be determined by the quantity of the drug involved; conspiracies and attempts to distribute marijuana are to be punished as severely as completed acts.

The United Nations (UN) International Conference on Drug Abuse and Illicit Trafficking recognizes that drug abuse is a global phenomenon affecting almost every country, although its extent and characteristics differ from region to region. At the time of the convention, the most widely consumed drug worldwide is cannabis. Three-quarters of all countries report abuse of heroin and two-thirds report abuse of cocaine. Drug-related problems include increased rates of crime and violence, susceptibility to HIV/AIDS and hepatitis, demand for treatment and emergency department visits, and a breakdown in social behavior.

At the 1988 UN General Assembly special session on the world drug problem, member states recognize that reducing the demand for drugs is an essential pillar in the stepped-up global effort to fight drug abuse and trafficking. Member states commit to reducing significantly both the supply of and demand for drugs by 2008.

1990 In *Smith v. Oregon*, the U.S. Supreme Court rules that the state could deny unemployment benefits to a person fired for violating a state prohibition on the use of peyote, even though the use of the drug was part of a religious ritual.

1992 The DEA administrator officially denies the petition of the NORML to reschedule marijuana from Schedule I to Schedule II of the Controlled Substances Act in 1989. On appeal, the decision is reviewed and the judicial decision is made that marijuana has no currently accepted medical use.

The DEA initiates the Kingpin Strategy to attack drug organizations at vulnerable areas—the chemicals needed to process the drugs, where they are made, and their finances, transportation, communications, and leadership infrastructure in the United States.

Manuel Noriega, the de facto leader of Panama and one-time operative for the Central Intelligence Agency, is captured and brought to the United States to stand trial. He is convicted on charges of racketeering, money laundering, and drug trafficking, and sentenced to 40 years in prison.

1996 Voters in California approve legislation, the Compassionate Use Act, Proposition 215, allowing sick and dying patients to use marijuana for medicinal purposes.

The Drug Free Communities Act becomes a catalyst for increased citizen participation in efforts to reduce substance abuse among youth and provide community antidrug coalitions with funds to carry out their missions.

Among the provisions, the Anti-Media Campaign is created as a government-funded initiative to reduce and prevent drug use among young people through the use of television, radio, and other advertising.

1997 The Children's Health Insurance Program Reauthorization Act authorizes expanded research and services for a variety of childhood health problems, reauthorizes programs of the Substance Abuse and Mental Health Services Administration, and addresses the problem of youth substance abuse and the violence associated with it. Other provisions include support for law enforcement to combat drugs such as methamphetamine and ecstasy. This legislation expands the Clinton administration's National Methamphetamine Strategy and efforts to reduce drug abuse through the Youth Anti-Drug Media Campaign.

2001 President Bush signs legislation, the Drug-Free Communities Act, to reduce the demand for illegal drugs through education, prevention, and treatment.

2002 Canada and England take legislative measures to lower penalties for cannabis use. A Canadian senate committee issues a white paper report recommending liberal cannabis legislation.

The U.S. Supreme Court rules, in *Board of Education of Independent School District No. 92 of Pottawatomie County v. Earls*, to allow drug testing of young people whom authorities have no particular reason to suspect of wrongdoing.

2003 The U.S. Government Accounting Office and other independent evaluators declare that major antidrug programs, such as the Drug Abuse Resistance Program, the National Youth Anti-Drug Media Campaign, and the DEA are failing to achieve measurable success objectives.

Representatives of 142 countries at the 46th session of the UN Commission on Narcotic Drugs in Vienna say they will stick to the strict policies established at a UN antidrug summit five years earlier despite critics' allegations that the program is ineffective. Participants say they remain committed to the campaign to curb cultivation, trafficking, and consumption by 2008.

President Bush announces a three-year, $600 million plan to help addicts receive treatment. The program will use vouchers that give addicts a way to pay for treatment services, including those provided by faith-based organizations.

Edward Rosenthal, a popular authority on marijuana, is arrested in Oakland, California, by DEA agents for distribution of marijuana for medical purposes under state law. Rosenthal is found guilty but is sentenced to one day and released. This arrest sets the stage for further judicial review regarding state and federal marijuana laws, jurisdiction, and enforcement.

The Illicit Drug Anti-Proliferation Act, formerly known as the RAVE Act, becomes law. This legislation makes it easier for prosecutors to charge, convict, and imprison property owners and business owners and managers who fail to prevent drug-related offenses committed by customers, employees, tenants, or other persons on their property. The law also authorizes funds to educate parents and children on the dangers of ecstasy and other predatory drugs, and it directs the U.S. Sentencing Commission to consider increasing sentencing penalties for offenses involving GHB, a drug used in sexual assaults.

Great Britain downgrades marijuana from a Class B to a Class C drug, putting it in the same category as bodybuilding steroids and certain antidepressants. Although the move is not considered a step toward legalization, the decriminalization bars British police from arresting people for using marijuana. Authorities argue that the downgrade will enable police to focus on harder drugs, such as heroin and crack cocaine, which cause more harm and crime.

2005 Tennessee becomes one of at least 22 states to enforce a tax on illegal drugs. Under the new law drug dealers will be required to pay excise taxes on illegal substances.

In *Gonzales v. Raich*, the U.S. Supreme Court holds that federal authorities may prosecute patients whose doctors prescribe medical marijuana despite state laws that allow its use.

The Federal Bureau of Investigation considers easing its ban on hiring applicants who admit to having used drugs, such as occasionally smoking marijuana in college. Current hiring standards bar applicants who used marijuana within the past three years or more than 15 times in their lifetime, or drugs such as cocaine and heroin within the past 10 years or more than five times in their lifetime.

The National Survey on Drug Use and Health reports that U.S. household residents are more likely to report nonmedical use of prescription drugs than the use of almost all illicit drugs. One in twenty persons 12 years or older report nonmedically using prescription pain relievers in the past year—more than any illicit drug with the exception of marijuana.

2007 Texas becomes the first state to require random testing of high school student athletes for steroids. New Jersey, the only other state to require steroid testing, screens high school athletes who make the playoffs. Federal studies indicate that around 2.7 percent of high school seniors have used steroids.

In *Morse v. Frederick*, the U.S. Supreme Court rules against a Juneau, Alaska, student who raised a banner with the words "Bong Hits for Jesus" at a school-sponsored event. In a 5–4 decision, the court rules that schools have the right to limit student speech that could be interpreted as advocating use of illicit drugs.

In *Kimbrough v. United States*, the U.S. Supreme Court upholds a judge's decision to violate federal sentencing guidelines and impose a shorter prison term than mandated on a man convicted of possession of crack cocaine. The court's ruling does not strike down the controversial law but rather empowers trial court judges to impose sentences below what the statutes proscribe. The day after this ruling, the U.S. Sentencing Commission, which has broad authority to set sentencing guidelines, makes retroactive an earlier decision that effectively eliminates the 100:1 imbalance. The commission's decision also means that some 2,500 convicted drug felons will be eligible for early release in 2008.

2008 The California State Supreme Court rules that employers can fire medical-marijuana users for violating workplace drug policies despite the fact that use of the drug is legal for medical purposes under state law.

President Bush requests $14.1 billion for the National Drug Control Budget in support of stopping drug use before it starts, healing America's drug users, and disrupting the market for illicit drugs. In 2002, the budget was $19.2 billion.

The executive director of the UN Office on Drugs and Crime, Antonio Maria Costa, reports to the 20th session of the General Assembly that in terms of annual prevalence, the drug control system has succeeded to contain drug problems to less than

5 percent of the adult population (aged 15–64) in the world. In comparative terms, he states that statistics point to an undeniable success. Unintended consequences are noted in his presentation relating to issues of a criminal black market, policy displacement, geographic displacement, substance displacement, and the way nations perceive and deal with users of illicit drugs (UNODC 2008).

The U.S Supreme Court declines to review a lower court decision that ordered Garden Grove, California, police to return marijuana seized from a medical marijuana patient. In November 2007, the California Fourth District Court of Appeal had ordered the marijuana returned, stating it is not the job of local police to enforce federal drug laws. The U.S. Supreme Court's refusal to review a lower court ruling is seen as a victory for medical marijuana advocates.

2009 President Obama names Seattle Police Chief Gil Kerlikowske to head the White House Office of National Drug Control Policy (ONDCP) in February; Thomas McClellan, one of the nation's leading drug and alcohol experts, is named Deputy Director in April.

The U.S. Supreme Court declares that Arizona school officials violated a 13-year-old girl's constitutional protection against unreasonable searches when they strip searched her on suspicion of possessing prescription-strength ibuprofen in violation of the school district's drug policy.

New York state legislators announce an agreement to dismantle the Rockefeller drug-sentencing laws—among the toughest in the nation—which were imposed during the heroin epidemic in the 1970s.

The U.S. Supreme Court turns down a San Diego County appeal that argued that the federal ban on medical marijuana supersedes state law. The decision means federal law does not preempt California's law, and local California officials must comply with state law.

President Obama signs the Family Smoking Prevention and Tobacco Control Act granting the Food and Drug Administration sweeping authority to regulate the manufacture, marketing, and sale of tobacco products. The Congressional Budget Office estimates that youth smoking will drop 11 percent over the next decade and adult smoking will drop by 2 percent.

The U.S. Supreme Court rules that crime-lab reports can no longer be used against defendants at trial unless the analyst who created the report testifies in court and is available for cross-examination. The decision expands the Sixth Amendment's confrontation clause that grants criminal defendants the right to be confronted with the witnesses against him.

The U.S. attorney general calls off prosecution of people who use marijuana for medical purposes and those who distribute it to them. In a Department of Justice memo, the importance of addressing criminal distribution and sale of marijuana, which is the largest source of revenue for the Mexican drug cartels is emphasized.

2010 ONDCP Deputy Director and his senior policy advisor announce their resignations effective in the summer of 2010.

ONDCP Director Kerlikowske announces that the Obama administration opposes legalizing marijuana before the 53rd United Nations Commission on Narcotic Drugs.

New Jersey joins 13 other states and the District of Columbia to make provisions for medical marijuana use.

California Proposition 19, also known as the Regulate, Control and Tax Cannabis Act of 2010, appeared as a statewide ballot on November 2. Rejected, the Act would have legalized various marijuana-related activities, allowed local governments to regulate such activities, collected marijuana-related fees and taxes, and authorized various criminal and civil penalties.

California Governor Arnold Schwarzenegger signs a bill, SB1449, to minimize the penalty of marijuana possession—up to an ounce is punishable by a $100 fine, but offenders would not be arrested or risk having a criminal record.

References

Brecher, E., and the editors of Consumer Reports. 1972. *Licit and Illicit Drugs: The Consumers Union Report on Narcotics, Stimulants Depressants, Inhalants, Hallucinogens, and Marijuana—including Caffeine, Nicotine, and Alcohol.* Boston: Little, Brown and Company.

Drug Enforcement Administration. 2010. DEA Mission Statement. Available at: http://www.justice.gov/dea/agency/mission.htm. Accessed October 2, 2010.

Schaffer Library on Drug Policy. 2010a. *Linder v. United States.* Available at: http://www.druglibrary.org/schaffer/history/1920.htm. Accessed September 16, 2010.

Schaffer Library on Drug Policy. 2010b. *NORML v. Bell et al.* Available at: http://www.druglibrary.org/Schaffer/legal/l1980/bell.htm. Accessed September 16, 2010.

United Nations Office on Drugs and Crime (UNODC). 2008. Annual Report 2008. Available at: http://www.unodc.org/documents/about-unodc/AR08_WEB.pdf. Accessed September 16, 2010.

U.S. House of Representatives, Select Committee on Narcotics Abuse and Control. 1978a. *Demand Reduction in the United States and Abroad* (SCNAC-95-2-11). Washington, D.C.: U.S. Government Printing Office.

U.S. House of Representatives, Select Committee on Narcotics Abuse and Control. 1978b. *Drug Abuse Treatment (Part 1)* (SCNAC-95-2-12). Washington, D.C.: U.S. Government Printing Office.

Woodward, W. 1937. American Medical Association Opposes the Marijuana Tax Act of 1937. Available at: http://www.marijuanalibrary.org/AMA_opposes_1937.html. Accessed September 16, 2010.

APPENDIX E

Directory of Organizations

The following agencies and organizations address drug issues from supply and demand control to legislation reform, prevention education, treatment and research. In addition, information is provided about significant nongovernment organizations, university-based research centers, and government organizations based in the United States.

GOVERNMENT AGENCIES

Centers for Disease Control and Prevention
1600 Clifton Road
Atlanta, GA 30333
800-CDC-INFO (800-232-4636) (toll-free phone)
E-mail: cdcinfo@cdc.gov
Web site: www.cdc.gov

National Clearinghouse for Alcohol and Drug Information (NCADI)
P.O. Box 2345
Rockville, MD 20847-2345
301-729-6686 (phone)
877-SAMHSA-7 (toll-free phone)
240-221-4292 (fax)
E-mail: webmaster@health.org
Web site: http://ncadi.samhsa.gov/

National Institute on Alcohol Abuse and Alcoholism (NIAAA)
5635 Fishers Lane, MSC 9304
Bethesda, MD 20892-9304
301-443-3860 (phone)
E-mail: niaaaweb-r@exchange.nih.gov
Web site: http://www.niaaa.nih.gov

National Institute on Drug Abuse (NIDA)
National Institutes of Health
6001 Executive Boulevard, Room 5213
Bethesda, MD 20892-9561
301-443-1124 (phone)
E-mail: Information@nida.nih.gov
Web site: http://www.nida.nih.gov

National Youth Anti-Drug Campaign
Drug Policy Information Clearinghouse
P.O. Box 6000
Bethesda, MD 20849-6000
800-666-3332 (toll-free phone)
301-519-5212 (fax)
E-mail: The site has an e-mail form.
Web site: www.whitehousedrugpolicy.gov/about/clearingh.html

Substance Abuse and Mental Health Services Administration (SAMHSA)
1 Choke Cherry Road
Rockville, MD 20857
877-726-4727 (toll-free phone)
240-221-4292 (fax)
E-mail: SHIN@samhsa.hhs.gov
Web site: http://www.samhsa.gov

Center for Substance Abuse Prevention (SAMSHA)
240-276-2420 (phone)
800-WORKPLACE (toll-free help line)
E-mail: info@samhsa.gov
Web site: http://prevention.samhsa.gov

Center for Substance Abuse Treatment (SAMSHA)
240-276-2750 (phone)
800-662-HELP (toll-free National Treatment Hotline)
E-mail: info@samhsa.gov
Web site: http://www.csat.samhsa.gov

White House Office of National Drug Control Policy (ONDCP)
Drug Policy Information Clearinghouse
P.O. Box 6000
Bethesda, MD 20849-6000
800-666-3332 (toll-free phone)
301-519-5212 (fax)

E-mail: The site has an e-mail form.
Web site: http://www.whitehousedrugpolicy.gov

Nongovernment Organizations (Selected Drug Organizations)

American Council for Drug Education
204 Monroe Street, Suite 110
Rockville, MD 20850
800-488-3784 (toll-free phone)
E-mail: acde@phoenixhouse.org
Web site: http://www.drughelp.org

Association for Medical Education and Research in Substance Abuse (AMERSA)
125 Whipple Street, 3rd Floor, Suite 300
Providence, RI 02908
401-243-8460 (phone)
877-418-8769 (toll-free phone)
Web site: http://www.amersa.org

College on Problems of Drug Dependence (CPDD)
3420 North Broad Street
Philadelphia, PA 19140
215-707-3242 (phone)
215-707-1904 (fax)
E-mail: baldeagl@temple.edu
Web site: http://www.cpdd.vcu.edu

Common Sense for Drug Policy
1377-C Spencer Ave.
Lancaster, PA 17603
717-299-0600 (phone)
717-393-4953 (fax)
Email: info@csdp.org
Web site: http://www.csdp.org

Community Anti-Drug Coalitions of America (CADCA)
625 Slaters Lane, Suite 300
Alexandria, VA 22314
800-54-CADCA (phone)
703-706-0565 (fax)
E-mail: The site has an e-mail form.
Web site: www.cadca.org

Drug Policy Alliance
70 West 36th Street, 16th Floor
New York, NY 10018
212-613-8020 (phone)
212-613-8021 (fax)
E-mail: nyc@drugpolicy.org
Web site: http://www.drugpolicy.org

Drug Abuse Resistance Education (D.A.R.E.)
9800 La Cienega Boulevard, Suite 401
Inglewood, CA 90301
800-223-DARE (toll-free phone) or 310-215-0575 (phone)
310-215-0108 (fax)
E-mail: The site has an e-mail form.
Web site: http://www.dare.com/home/default.asp

Drug Reform Coordination Network
1623 Connecticut Avenue NW, 3rd Floor
Washington, DC 20009
202-293-8340 (phone)
202-293-8344 (fax)
E-mail: drcnet@drcnet.org
Web site: http://www.drcnet.org/aboutdrc/

Drug Strategies
800-559-9503 (toll-free hotline phone)
E-mail: dspolicy@aol.com
Web site: www.drugstrategies.org

Drug Watch International
P.O. Box 45218
Omaha, NE 68145-0218
402-384-9212 (phone)
Web site: http://www.drugwatch.org

Foundation for a Drug-Free World
1626 North Wilcox Avenue, Suite 1297
Los Angeles, CA 90028
888-668-6378 (toll-free phone)
E-mail: info@drugfreeworld.org
Web Site: http://www.drugfreeworld.org/activities/index.html

Hazelden Foundation
P. O. Box 11
Center City, MN 55012-0011

800-257-7810 (toll-free helpline phone)
E-mail: info@hazelden.org
Web site: http://www.hazelden.org

Join Together
715 Albany Street, 580–3rd floor
Boston, MA 02118
617-437-1500 (phone)
617-437-9394 (fax)
E-mail: info@jointogether.org
Web site: http://www.jointogether.org/

National Council on Alcoholism and Drug Dependence (NCADD)
244 East 58th Street, 4th Floor
New York, NY 10005
800-NCA-CALL (toll-free hotline)
212-269-7797 (phone)
212-269-7510 (fax)
E-mail: national@ncadd.org
Web site: http://www.ncadd.org

National Organization of Reform for Marijuana Laws (NORML)
1600 K Street NW, Suite 501
Washington, DC 20006-2832
888-67-NORML (toll-free phone)
202-483-5500 (phone)
202-483-0057 (fax)
E-mail: norml@norml.org
Web site: http://www.norml.org

Partnership for a Drug Free America (PDFA)
405 Lexington Avenue, Suite 1601
New York, NY 10174
212-922-1560 (phone)
212-922-1570 (fax)
E-mail: The site has an e-mail form.
Web site: www.drugfree.org

Robert Wood Johnson Foundation—Substance Abuse Policy Research Program
One Leadership Place
Greensboro, NC 27410
336-286-4548 (phone)
336-286-4434 (fax)
Web site: http://www.saprp.org/p_natProg.cfm

University-Based Drug Research and Policy Centers

National Center on Addiction and Substance Abuse at Columbia University (CASA)
633 Third Avenue, Floor 19
New York, NY 10017-6706
212-841-5200 (phone)
Web site: http://www.casacolumbia.org

Monitoring the Future Study, University of Michigan
University of Michigan
Ann Arbor, MI 48109
E-mail: MTFinfo@isr.umich.edu
Web site: http://monitoringthefuture.org/

University of California, Integrated Substance Abuse Programs (ISAP)
11075 Santa Monica Boulevard, Suite 200
Los Angeles, CA 90025
310-312-0500, ext. 317 (phone)
E-mail: darc@ucla.edu
Web site: http://www.uclaisap.org

University of Kentucky Center on Drug and Alcohol Research (CDAR)
643 Maxwelton Court
Lexington, KY 40506-0350
859-257-2355 (phone)
859-323-1193 (fax)
E-mail: krieger@uky.edu
Web site: http://cdar.uky.edu/

University of Maryland—Center for Substance Abuse Research (CESAR)
4321 Hartwick Road, Suite 501
College Park, MD 20740
301-403-8329 (phone)
301-403-8342 (fax)
E-mail: cesar@cesar.umd.edu
Web site: http://www.cesar.umd.edu

Glossary

Abstinence This is the conscious choice not to use drugs. The term "abstinence" usually refers to the decision to end the use of a drug as part of the process of recovery from addiction.

Abuse A term with a range of meanings. In international drug control conventions "abuse" refer to any consumption of a controlled substance no matter how infrequent (*see also* drug abuse).

Acetaminophen A common analgesic and anti-fever drug with no psychoactive properties, frequently found in combination with opiate pain killers in prescription form.

Acute A sharp, rapid, or short-term episode or effect, as opposed to a chronic or long-term condition, use, or effect.

Adaptive behaviors Useful behaviors people acquire as they respond to the world around them. Adaptive behaviors help people get the things they want and need for life.

Addiction A brain disorder characterized by the loss of control of drug-taking behavior, despite adverse health, social, or legal consequences to continued drug use. Addiction tends to be chronic and tends to be characterized by relapses during recovery; a chronic, relapsing disease.

Addictive drug A drug that changes the brain, changes behavior, and leads to the loss of control of drug-taking behavior.

Agonist A chemical that mimics or facilitates the effects of a neurotransmitter.

Alcohol The world's most popular drug, legally used in most countries. Alcohol is produced through the fermentation of fruits, vegetables, and grains.

Alcoholics Anonymous One of the earliest methods of addiction treatment in the United States, Alcoholics Anonymous, or AA, developed the 12-step approach to assisting recovery from alcohol addiction (alcoholism). Several other anonymous groups have adapted the 12-step approach to help people recover from addiction to other drugs (e.g., Narcotics Anonymous, Cocaine Anonymous, Pot Smokers Anonymous).

Alveoli Tiny, balloon-like air sacks in the lungs. Alveoli are designed to allow oxygen to pass rapidly into the blood and are efficient at absorbing inhaled drugs, such as crack cocaine.

Amotivational syndrome A constellation of effects said to be associated with substance use (especially of cannabis), including apathy, loss of effectiveness, diminished capacity to carry out complex or long-term plans, low tolerance for frustration, impaired concentration, and difficulty following routines.

Amphetamine Stimulant drug whose effects are very similar to cocaine. Often called "speed," this drug is a synthetically produced central nervous system stimulant with cocaine-like effects.

Analgesic A substance that reduces pain and may or may not have psychoactive properties.

Angel Dust Street term for phencyclidine (PCP), a dissociative hallucinogen.

Anhedonia Inability to feel pleasure in activities usually enjoyed. Found in many drug withdrawal states, as well as in depression and schizophrenia.

Antagonist A substance (e.g., naloxone) that counteracts the effects of another agent (e.g., opiate drug).

Anxiolytic Anti-anxiety drug, which may include any of the minor tranquilizers, such as the benzodiazepines.

Barbiturate Depressant drugs that produce relaxation and sleep. Barbiturates include sleeping pills such as pentobarbital (Nembutal) and secobarbital (Seconal).

Behavioral tolerance Where a drug user learns to compensate for the effects of a drug, such as learning to walk in a straight line while under the influence of a depressant.

Benzodiazepine Any of a group of depressants known as minor tranquilizers that relieve anxiety and produce sleep. Benzodiazepines include tranquilizers, such as diazepam (Valium) and alprazolam (Xanax), and sleeping pills, such as flurazepam (Dalmane) and triazolam (Halcion).

Binge Uninterrupted consumption of a drug for several hours or days.

Black tar Street term for a powerful form of heroin.

Brief intervention A treatment strategy in which structured therapy of a limited number of sessions (usually one to four) of short duration (typically 5 to

30 minutes) is offered with the aim of helping a person cease or reduce the use of a psychoactive substance or to deal with other life issues.

Buprenorphine A long-lasting opiate analgesic that has both opiate agonist and antagonist properties. Buprenorphine shows promise for treating heroin addiction.

Caffeine A mild stimulant, the most widely used drug in the world.

Cannabinoid receptor The receptor in the brain that recognizes THC (tetrahydrocannabinol), the active ingredient in marijuana. Marijuana exerts its psychoactive effects via this receptor.

Cannabis The botanical name for the plant from which marijuana comes.

Central nervous system (CNS) The brain and spinal cord.

Chronic Long-term, persistent use or effects. Addiction is considered to be a chronic disorder in that its symptoms may persist and flare up despite short-term treatment.

Cocaine A bitter, crystalline drug obtained from the dried leaves of the coca shrub; it is a local anesthetic and a dangerous, illegal stimulant; it is the primary psychoactive ingredient in the coca plant and a behavioral-affecting drug.

Coca paste (or cocaine base) An extract of the coca bush leaves. Purification of coca paste yields cocaine.

Codeine A natural opioid compound that is a relatively weak, but still effective, opiate analgesic. It has also been used to treat other problems (e.g., to relieve coughing).

Controlled substance A term that refers to a psychoactive substance and its precursors whose availability is forbidden under the international drug control treaties or limited to medical and pharmaceutical channels.

Crack cocaine Cocaine base obtained from cocaine hydrochloride through conversion processes to make it suitable for smoking.

Craving hunger for drugs This condition is caused by drug-induced changes that occur in the brain with the development of addiction and arises from the brain's need to maintain a state of homeostasis that includes the presence of the drug.

Cross-dependence Where administration of a drug prevents withdrawal symptoms from another, similar drug.

Cross-tolerance Where tolerance to a drug results in tolerance or diminished effects of other, similar drugs.

Cutting agent A powder used to dilute cocaine, heroin, and other drugs used in powder form. Lactose (i.e., "milk sugar") and mannitol are examples.

D.A.R.E. (Drug Abuse Resistance Education) A school-based drug prevention program using local police officers as educators.

Date-rape drug A drug used by a sexual predator to induce sedation or sleep in their victim.

Demand reduction This approach reflects the policy that reducing the supply and availability of illicit drugs is an essential component of the fight against drug abuse. Efforts to limit the cultivation, production, trafficking, and distribution of drugs are strategies to implement this approach. Supply-reduction projects also seek to broaden regional cooperation between governments in response to cross-border trafficking, strengthen border controls by providing modern equipment, and develop training in best-practice law enforcement procedures.

Depressants drug A drug that relieves anxiety and produces sleep. Depressants include barbiturates, benzodiazepines, and alcohol.

Designer drug An illegally manufactured chemical whose molecular structure is altered slightly from a parent compound to enhance specific effects. Examples include DMT, DMA, DOM, MDA, and MDMA (ecstasy).

Detoxification The process of removing a drug from the body. This is the initial period addicts must go through to become drug-free. Withdrawal symptoms appear early during this process. Depending on the drug, detoxification lasts for a few days to a week or more.

Diversion Taking legally prescribed medications (e.g., methadone, tranquilizers) and selling them illegally. The term is also used to mean the provision of activities that move a person away from drug use.

Downer Street term for a depressant drug, usually a sedative such as barbiturates.

Drug A term of varied usage. In various United Nations conventions and in the Declaration of Drug Demand Reduction, it refers to substances subject to international control. In medicine, it refers to any substance with the potential to prevent or cure disease or enhance physical or mental well-being. In pharmacology, it refers to any chemical agent that alters the biochemical or psychological processes of tissues or organisms. In common usage, the term often refers specifically to psychoactive drugs, and often, even more specifically, to illicit drugs.

Drug abuse Using illegal drugs or using legal drugs inappropriately; the repeated, high-dose, self-administration of drugs to produce pleasure, alleviate stress, or alter or avoid reality (or all three).

Drug court Special court set up to divert drug offenders from the criminal justice system into treatment programs.

Drug dependence Compulsive use of a drug, loss of control over use, and inability to abstain. Similar to *drug addiction.*

Drug-free treatment Approaches to helping addicts recover from addiction without the use of medication.

Drug treatment A combination of detoxification, psychosocial therapy, and, if required, skill acquisition to help people recover from addiction.

Dual diagnosis (comorbidity) A person diagnosed as having an alcohol or drug abuse problem in addition to some other diagnosis, usually psychiatric (e.g., mood disorder, schizophrenia).

Ecstasy (MDMA or 3,4-methylenedioxymethamphetamine) A chemically modified amphetamine that has hallucinogenic and stimulant properties. Also called "E," "XTC," and "Adam."

Effective dose Dose of a drug that produces a certain effect in a given percentage of subjects, often half of the subjects to whom the drug is administered.

Ephedra A plant genus comprising some 40 distinct species that grow wild in various regions of the world. Ephedra has a long history of medical and ceremonial purposes. Ephedra contains two principle alkaloids, ephedrine and pseudoephedrine, which are used in medicines worldwide.

FDA U.S. Food and Drug Administration. FDA is an agency within the Department of Health and Human Services. It is responsible for protecting the public health by assuring the safety, efficacy, and security of human and veterinary drugs, biological products, medical devices, the nation's food supply, cosmetics, and products that emit radiation, and by regulating the manufacture, marketing, and distribution of tobacco products.

Freebase cocaine Where cocaine hydrochloride is separated from its hydrochloride base, which is volatile and smokable.

Gateway theory A model of the progression of drug use that has grown out of research with adolescents that has identified a sequential pattern of involvement in various legal and illegal drugs.

Generic name The common name of a drug, such as acetaminophen, as opposed to a brand or proprietary name, such as Tylenol.

GHB (gamma hydroxybutyrate) Originally developed as an anesthetic but was withdrawn because of unwanted side effects. At small doses, GHB tends to reduce social inhibitions, similar in action to alcohol; it is also reported to increase libido.

Half-life The time during which half of a given drug is eliminated from the body.

Hallucinogen Any of a diverse group of drugs that alter perceptions, thoughts, and feelings. Hallucinogens do not produce hallucinations. These drugs include LSD, mescaline, MDMA (ecstasy), PCP, and psilocybin (magic mushrooms).

Harm reduction A set of practical strategies that reduce negative consequences of drug use by incorporating a range of strategies from safer use to managed use to abstinence. Because harm reduction demands that interventions and policies designed to serve drug users reflect specific individual and community needs, there is no universal definition of or formula for implementing it.

Hashish Cannabis preparation more potent than marijuana. This comes from the resinous secretions of the marijuana plant's flowering tops.

Hemp The marijuana plant, usually referring to plants harvested for fiber.

Heroin (diacetylmorphine) The potent, widely abused opiate that produces a profound addiction. Heroin no.3 is a less refined form of heroin suitable for smoking. Originally a trade name of Bayer Pharmaceuticals.

Huff Slang term for the inhalation of a volatile, psychoactive substance, such as when airplane glue is concentrated in a bag before breathing in.

Hydrocodone A semi-synthetic opioid; it is a narcotic used to relieve pain; it produces a calm, euphoric state similar to heroin or morphine. This drug is stronger than codeine, but about one-tenth as potent as morphine. It is often used in combination with acetaminophen, aspirin, or ibuprofen. Hydrocodone addiction is a growing crisis in the United States.

Hypnotic Sleep inducing.

Ice A smokable form of methamphetamine. By smoking the drug it affects the body more quickly.

Inhalant Any drug administered by breathing in its vapors. This category includes psychoactive nonpharmaceutical substances and anesthetic gases for which the documented route of administration is inhalation, sniffing, or snorting. Inhaled substances fall into one of the following three categories: (1) volatile solvent—adhesives, aerosols, gases, cleaning agents, food products; (2) nitrite (amyl nitrite—"poppers" used for recreational purposes and air fresheners); or (3) chlorofluorohydrocarbon (freons). These substances are very dangerous and are often used by young people.

Intoxication Being under the influence of, and responding to, the acute effects of a psychoactive drug. Intoxication typically includes feelings of pleasure, altered emotional responsiveness, altered perception, and impaired judgment and performance.

Intranasal administration Snorting a drug into the nasal passage, where it is absorbed into the mucous membranes.

Intravenous (IV) A method of injecting a drug into a vein.

Khat The leaves and buds of an East African plant used to suppress appetite and combat fatigue. It is a controlled/illegal substance in many countries; it induces mild euphoria and hyperactivity.

LAAM (levo-alpha-acetyl methadol) A very long-lasting opiate agonist recently approved for the treatment of opiate addiction.

LD (lethal dose) The amount of a drug that causes death in a specified proportion of subjects, often one-half of the population, expressed as LD50.

Long-term effects The effects seen when a drug is used repeatedly over weeks, months, or years. These effects may outlast drug use.

LSD (d-lysergic acid diethylamide) This chemical was synthesized from ergot in 1938 by Albert Hofmann of the Sandoz Laboratories in Switzerland; a powerful hallucinogen whose effective dose is 200 to 400 micrograms, a mere speck in size.

Marijuana The *Cannabis sativa* plant that produces a mild euphoric effect. The active ingredient that produces the euphoric effect is THC (tetrahydrocannabinol). Marijuana can be eaten or smoked in cigarette form or pipes. The oily resin of the marijuana plant can be used to produce hashish or hashish oil.

Marinol The trade name of dronabinol, a synthetic version of THC used as medicine.

MDMA (ecstasy) 3,4-Methylenedioxymethamphetamine. A hallucinogenic designer drug with psychedelic and stimulant properties.

Mescaline A naturally occurring hallucinogenic drug found in the peyote cactus. Mescaline is not found in the mescal cactus from which tequila is acquired.

Methadone A long-lasting synthetic opiate used to treat cancer pain and heroin addiction. Methadone use can be addictive.

Methamphetamine A commonly abused, potent stimulant drug that is part of a larger family of amphetamines.

Methylphenidate An amphetamine-like drug used to medicate attention-deficit hyperactivity disorder, marketed as Ritalin.

Morphine A powerful narcotic that comes from the opium plant. Heroin is derived from morphine. It is named after the Greek god Morpheus, the god of sleep.

Motivational interviewing A counseling and assessment technique that uses a nonconfrontational approach to questioning people about difficult issues like alcohol and other drug use and helps them to make positive decisions to reduce or stop their drug use altogether.

Naloxone A short-acting opiate antagonist that binds to and blocks opiate receptors, preventing opiates from binding to these receptors. Naloxone is used to treat opiate overdoses.

Narcotic Addictive opiate or synthetic opiate with powerful pain-killing properties.

Narcotics Anonymous A peer-led self-help fellowship of recovering addicts, based on the 12-step model pioneered by Alcoholics Anonymous.

Neurotransmitter Chemical messenger released between nerve cells in the central nervous system.

Nicotine The addictive drug in tobacco. Nicotine also activates a specific kind of acetylcholine receptor.

Nicotine gum, nicotine patch Two methods of delivering small amounts of nicotine into the bodies of people who are addicted to nicotine to help them quit smoking cigarettes by preventing nicotine withdrawal.

NIDA (National Institute of Drug Abuse) NIDA focuses on key issues about drug abuse, ranging from the molecule to managed care to DNA to community outreach research.

Opiate Any of the psychoactive drugs that originate from the opium poppy or that have a chemical structure like the drugs derived from opium. Such drugs include opium, codeine, and morphine, which are derived from the plant, and hydromorphone (Dilaudid), methadone, and meperidine (Demerol), which were first synthesized by chemists.

Opioid Any chemical that has opiate-like effects; commonly used to refer to endogenous neurochemicals that activate opiate receptors.

Opioid antagonist Drug that blocks the effects of opioids; used to treat overdose or prevent abuse; examples include nalorphine and naltrexone.

Opium The milky latex fluid that comes from the seed pod of the opium poppy. When the fluid is drawn from the pod, it turns black and hardens into a form in which it can be smoked. Opium is highly addictive and has been used for centuries for medicinal purposes and/or to achieve a sense of euphoria, calm, and well-being.

OTC drug (over-the-counter drug) A drug available without a prescription.

Outpatient treatment Nonresidential treatment for drug addiction. Patients live at home, often work, and go to a clinic for treatment.

Overdose The condition that results when too much of a drug is taken, making a person sick or unconscious and sometimes resulting in death.

OxyContin An opiate derivative intended for use by pain sufferers and terminal cancer patients. It is a time-released form of oxycodone. Addiction and abuse, including fatal overdoses, of the drug is a growing problem.

Papaver somniferum Genus and species for the opium poppy.

Paranoid schizophrenia A severe form of mental illness characterized by delusions of persecution and hallucinations. Binge use of stimulants may produce a temporary psychotic condition that resembles paranoid schizophrenia.

PCP (phencyclidine) Originally developed as an anesthetic, PCP may act as a hallucinogen, stimulant, or sedative.

Percocet A narcotic (oxycodone) and acetaminophen (e.g., Tylenol) combination used for pain control. This drug is addictive.

Percodan Like Percocet, this drug is a combination of oxycodone and aspirin.

Persian heroin Heroin in a smokable form. Smoking heroin is often called "chasing the dragon."

Peyote The cactus that contains the hallucinogenic chemical mescaline.

Poppy straw All parts (except the seeds) of the opium poppy left after mowing.

Prevention Stopping drug use before it starts, intervening to halt the progression of drug use once it has begun, or changing environmental conditions that encourage addictive drug use.

Primary reinforcer Stimulus, such as food and water, that produces reward directly, with no learning about their significance or other intervening steps required. Most drugs of abuse are primary reinforcers.

Psilocybe Often referred to as "magic mushrooms," this genus of fungus contains two hallucinogens—psilocybin and psilocin. There are a number of other poisonous and hallucinogenic mushrooms.

Psilocybin A natural hallucinogenic drug derived from a mushroom that acts on the serotonin receptor.

Psychedelic drug Drug that distorts perception, thought, and feeling. This term is typically used to refer to drugs with actions like those of LSD.

Psychoactive drug A drug that changes the way the brain works.

Psychological dependence When drugs become so central to a user's life that the user believes he must use them.

Psychopharmacology Scientific field that studies and describes the effects of drugs on the mind and behavior.

Psychosis Severe mental illnesses characterized by loss of contact with reality. Schizophrenia and severe depression are psychoses.

Psychosocial therapy Therapy designed to help addicts by using a combination of individual psychotherapy and group (social) therapy approaches to rehabilitate or provide the interpersonal and intrapersonal skills needed to live without drugs.

Rapid assessment A variety of methods for rapid or focused data collection that since the 1980s have grown out of a sense of urgency for social science input in disease-control programs.

Rehabilitate Helping a person recover from drug addiction. Rehabilitation teaches the addict new behaviors to live life without drugs.

Relapse In general, to fall back to a former condition. With substance abuse, resuming the use of a drug one has tried to stop using. Relapse is a common occurrence in many chronic disorders that require behavioral adjustments to treat effectively.

REM rebound In stopping the chronic use of a depressant, there may be an increase in vivid, even frightening "dream sleep" also known as REM for "rapid eye movement."

Residential treatment Treatment program that requires participants to live in a hostel, home, residential hall, or hospital unit.

Reward The process that reinforces behavior.

Risk reduction Describes policies or programs that focus on reducing the risk of harm from alcohol or other drug use.

Ritalin Trade name for methylphenidate, a central nervous system stimulant. More potent than caffeine but less potent than amphetamines, this drug is often prescribed for children and youth believed to have attention-deficit hyperactivity disorder. Like other stimulants, it is addictive and has a high potential for abuse.

Rock A small amount of crack cocaine in a solid form; free-base cocaine in solid form.

Route of administration The way a drug is put into the body. Eating, drinking, inhaling, injecting, snorting, smoking, and absorbing a drug through mucous membranes are all routes of administration used to consume drugs of abuse.

Run A binge of (more or less) uninterrupted consumption of a drug for several hours or days. This pattern of drug use is typically associated with stimulants but is also seen with alcohol.

Rush Intense feelings of euphoria a drug produces when first consumed. Drug users who inject or smoke drugs describe the rush as being sometimes as intense, or even more intense, than sexual orgasm.

SAMHSA (Substance Abuse and Mental Health Services Administration) A federal agency involved with study, treatment research, and information dissemination related to alcohol, drug, and psychiatric disorders.

Seconal A depressant drug of the barbiturate family that induces sleep.

Sedative/hypnotic Any of a group of central nervous system depressants with the capacity of relieving anxiety and inducing calmness and sleep.

Sinsemilla Marijuana grown without allowing the female plants to be pollinated; this means the flowers, which contain the highest concentration of THC, cluster and excrete greater quantities of resin. Sinsemilla means "no seeds."

Skin popping Injecting a drug under the skin.

Snowballing A method of recruiting illicit drug users for research purposes or peer-based prevention purposes.

Stimulant A class of drugs that elevates mood, increases feelings of well-being, and increases energy and alertness. These drugs also produce euphoria and are powerfully rewarding. Stimulants include cocaine, methamphetamine, and methylphenidate (Ritalin).

STP This synthetically produced hallucinogen is a variation of mescaline and amphetamines. It is generally less potent than LSD but takes longer to break down in the body; therefore, it lasts much longer, in some instances 24 hours to several days.

Supply reduction A broad term used for a range of activities designed to stop the production, manufacture, and distribution of illegal drugs. Production can be curtailed through crop eradication or large programs of alternative development.

Synergistic effect Where two drugs are taken together so they multiply each other's effects; this has the potential for a toxic or lethal effect.

Synesthesia While using a hallucinogen, sensory information may cross over into another sensory system, so that a user may "hear" colors or "see" music.

THC (tetrahydrocannabinol) The active ingredient in marijuana.

Therapeutic community Community that provides long-term, residential treatment for drug addiction, offering detoxification, group therapy, and skill acquisition.

Therapeutic window or therapeutic index Margin of safety between a dose that produces the intended effect and the dose that causes death, often expressed as a ratio (lethal dose/effective dose).

Tolerance A physiological change resulting from repeated drug use that requires the user to consume increasing amounts of the drug to get the same effect a smaller dose used to give.

Tranquilizer Depressant drug that relieves anxiety and produce sedation.

Transdermal absorption Absorption through the skin.

Trigger Formerly neutral stimuli that have attained the ability to elicit drug craving after repeated pairing with drug use; also called "cues."

12-step group A mutual-help group organized around the 12-step program of Alcoholics Anonymous or a close adaptation of that program.

Valium A depressant drug of the benzodiazepine family that relieves anxiety.

Vicodin An opium derivative that is a commonly prescribed and abused prescription pain medication. Vicodin can cause depression and can affect thought processes, attention and judgment.

Withdrawal Physical symptoms in the body and brain that occur after a person who is physically dependent on that drug ceases its use.

Xanax (aprazalom) A depressant drug of the benzodiazepine family that relieves anxiety.

Further Reading

Select Books

The authors of this volume recommend the following books for further research. The annotations are quoted or summarized from the publishers' descriptions of the books. (A comprehensive listing of books addressing illicit drug issues is available from the Substance Abuse Librarians and Information Specialists (SALIS) Web site at http://salis.org/resources/newbooks_archive_current.htm#A.)

Brady, K. T., S. E. Back, and S. F. Greenfield, eds. 2009. *Women and Addiction: A Comprehensive Handbook.* New York: Guilford Press.
Scientific awareness of sex and gender differences in substance use disorders has grown tremendously in recent decades. This volume brings together leading authorities to review the state of the science and identify key directions for research and clinical practice.

Briggs, C. A., and J. L. Pepperell. 2009. *Women, Girls, and Addiction: Celebrating the Feminine in Counseling Treatment and Recovery*. Routledge.
This is the first book on the efficacy of treatment approaches and interventions that are tailored to working with addicted women, and the first publication of any kind to provide a feminist approach to understanding the experience of addiction from the female perspective.

Cohen, L. M., F. L. Collins Jr., A. Young, D. E. McChargue, T. R. Leffingwell, and K. L. Cook, eds. 2009. *Pharmacology and Treatment of Substance Abuse: Evidence and Outcome Based Perspectives.* Routledge.
Given the prevalence of substance abuse in general clinical populations, it is important for health care providers to have knowledge and skill in the treatment of these problems. Evidence-based practice involves the integration of the best evidence with clinical expertise and patient values.

Copello, A., J. Orford, R. Hodgson, and G. Tober. 2009. *Social Behaviour and Network Therapy for Alcohol Problems.* Routledge.
This book serves as a manual for clinicians working with people with alcohol problems. It is based on previous research in addiction treatment, including family and social network interventions, and the authors' own work developing and evaluating social behavior and network therapy.

Cupit Swenson, C., S. W. Henggeler, I. S. Taylor, and O. W. Addison. 2009. *Multisystemic Therapy and Neighborhood Partnerships: Reducing Adolescent Violence and Substance Abuse.* Guilford Press.
Based on the proven technology of multisystemic therapy, this unique book provides an exemplary approach to empowering communities to reduce youth violence and substance abuse and promote school success. Effective strategies for working with at-risk youth are embedded in a comprehensive framework that enlists the talents and resources of clinicians, human service professionals, neighborhood residents, community organizations, and outside stakeholders.

Fisher G., and N. Roget, eds. 2008. *Encyclopedia of Substance Abuse Prevention, Treatment, and Recovery.* Sage.
This work presents state-of-the-art research and evidence-based applications in approximately 350 signed entries that focus on the information addiction treatment and prevention and allied health professionals need to effectively work with clients.

Hart, K., C. Ksir, and O. Ray. 2008. *Drugs, Society, and Human Behavior.* 13th ed. McGraw-Hill.
Designed for an introduction to drugs and substance abuse course as taught in departments of health education, psychology, biology, sociology, and criminal justice, this full-color market-leading text provides the latest information on drug use and its effects on society and human behavior.

Inciardi, J. A., and K. McElrath, eds. 2007. *The American Drug Scene: An Anthology.* Oxford University Press.
The anthology is a collection of contemporary and classic articles on the changing patterns, problems, perspectives, and policies of legal and illicit drug use. The editors focus on the social contexts in which drug usage, drug-related problems, and drug policies occur.

Karch, S. 2006. *Drug Abuse Handbook.* 2nd ed. CRC Press.
This handbook is a thorough compendium of the knowledge of the pharmacological, medical, and legal aspects of drugs. The book examines criminalistics, pathology, pharmacokinetics, neurochemistry, treatment, as well as the ethical, legal, and practical issues involved with drugs and drug testing in the workplace and sports.

Korsmeyer, P., and H. Kranzler, eds. 2008. *Encyclopedia of Drugs, Alcohol & Addictive Behavior.* 3rd ed. Gale.

The encyclopedia is a multidisciplinary work with signed articles by respected scholars from international research centers. Volume one has a list of the editors and contributors and a table of contents for the entire set. The alphabetically arranged articles are two- to four-pages long and cover psychology, pharmacology, countries, organizations, and legal issues.

Lowinson, J., P. Ruiz, R. Millman, and J. Langrod. 2004. *Substance Abuse. A Comprehensive Textbook.* 4th ed. Lippincott Williams & Wilkins.
The updated and expanded 4th edition on substance abuse and addictive behaviors contains insights from more than 150 experts of patient management and research. This edition features coverage of the neurobiology of abused substances, new pharmacologic therapies for addictions, and complete information on club drugs such as ecstasy. Sections focus on addiction in children, adolescents, adults, and the elderly and women's health issues, including pregnancy. The behavioral addictions section includes hoarding, shopping, and computer/Internet abuse.

Mosher, C. J., and S. M. Akins. 2006. *Drugs and Drug Policy: The Control of Consciousness Alteration.* Sage.
This book provides a cross-national perspective on the regulation of drug use by examining and critiquing drug policies in the United States and abroad in terms of scope, goals, and effectiveness. The authors discuss the physiological, psychological, and behavioral effects of legal and illicit drugs; patterns and correlates of use; and theories on causes of drug use.

Musto, D. 2002. *Drugs in America: A Documentary History*. NYU Press.
In the first anthology of its kind, renowned drug policy expert David Musto chronicles the rise and fall and rise again of the most popular mind-altering substances in the United States: alcohol, marijuana, cocaine, and opiates.

Roll, J. M., R. A. Rawson, W. Ling, and S. Shoptaw, eds. 2009. *Methamphetamine Addiction: From Basic Science to Treatment*. Guilford Press.
Separating myth from fact, this authoritative work reviews the breadth of current knowledge about methamphetamine addiction and describes the most promising available treatment approaches. Leading experts present state-of-the-art information on the effects of methamphetamine on the brain, the body, and users' mental health and behavior.

Stimmel, B. 1996. *Drug Abuse and Social Policy in America: The War That Must Be Won (Haworth Therapy for the Addictive Disorders)*. Routledge.
A comprehensive text with an instructor's manual, *Drug Abuse and Social Policy in America* analyzes why current U.S. policy on the use of licit and illicit mood-altering drugs has failed. This groundbreaking book addresses differences between decriminalization, legalization, and zero tolerance—areas and philosophies that are poorly understood—and suggests a multipronged approach to diminish inappropriate drug use.

Straussner, L., and S. Brown, eds. 2000. *The Handbook of Addiction Treatment for Women.* Jossey-Bass.
This edited book addresses the special needs of women who are addicted to drugs, alcohol, and other self-destructive behaviors.

Sussman, S., and S. Ames. 2008. *Drug Abuse: Concepts, Prevention and Cessation.* Cambridge University Press.
This book is a comprehensive source of information on the topography of, causes of, and solutions to drug problems. The text covers conceptual issues regarding definitions of drug use, misuse, abuse, and dependence. It also addresses a variety of theoretical bases currently applied to the development of prevention and cessation programs, specific program content from evidence-based programs, and program processes and modalities.

United Nations. 2008. *Precursors and Chemicals Frequently Used in the Illicit Manufacture of Narcotic Drugs and Psychotropic Substances 2007.* United Nations.
To prevent the diversion of precursor chemicals for use in the illicit manufacture of drugs, governments must have adequate legislation in line with the United Nations Convention against Illicit Traffic in Narcotic Drugs and Psychotropic Substances. The International Narcotics Control Board, in its annual report, examines actions taken recently and highlights both successful results and shortcomings.

Walker, I. 2007. *Steroids: Pumped Up and Dangerous (Illicit and Misused Drugs).* Mason Crest Publishers.
Geared to high school athletes, this book reveals the dangerous side effects of steroids, both short and long term and examines treatment for and the legal consequences of using illegal steroids.

Noteworthy Drug Journals and Newsletters

The following list includes journals and newsletters devoted to topics related to illicit drugs. For most titles, the publication's scope, author guidelines, table of contents, and subscription information are presented. A few journals provide the full text of articles online. Each journal and newsletter has been checked for an active Web site. These references have been drawn from the ATOD Serials Database maintained by Nancy Sutherland, Meg Brunner, and Pam Miles, of the University of Washington Alcohol & Drug Abuse Institute Library. The database may be accessed through the SALIS Web site (http://lib.adai.washington.edu/salisserials.htm).

Addiction. Table of Contents (TOC), subscription information, instructions for contributors. (www.addictionjournal.org)

Addiction Abstracts. TOC, subscription information. (www.tandf.co.uk/addiction-abs)

Addiction Biology. TOC, subscription information, and instructions for contributors. (http://www.wiley.com/bw/journal.asp?ref=1355–6215)

Addiction Research and Theory. Aims and scope, instructions for authors, and subscription information. (www.tandf.co.uk/journals/titles/16066359.html)

Addiction Treatment Forum. Newsletter; full text. (www.atforum.com)

The Addictions Newsletter. From the American Psychological Association. (http://www.apa.org/divisions/div50/newsletter.htm)

Addictive Behaviors. TOC, guide for authors, order information. (http://www.elsevier.com/wps/find/journaldescription.cws_home/471/description#description)

Adicciones. Published by Socidrogalcohol, this quarterly journal on alcohol and other drug problems is widely distributed in Spanish-speaking countries; online abstracts in Spanish and English. (www.adicciones.org)

Alcohol, Tobacco, and Other Drugs Section Newsletter. Newsletter of American Public Health Assoc. ATOD section. (http://www.apha.org/membergroups/sections/aphasections/atod/)

American Indian and Alaska Native Mental Health Research. Journal of the National Center for American Indian and Alaska Native Mental Health Research, University of Colorado. (http://aianp.uchsc.edu/ncaianmhr/journal_home.htm)

American Journal on Addictions. American Psychiatric Association. TOC, author instructions, order information. (www.tandf.co.uk/journals/titles/10550496.html)

American Journal of Drug and Alcohol Abuse. TOC with abstracts, author guidelines, editorial scope, order information. (http://www.informaworld.com/smpp/title~content=t713597226~db=all)

Drug and Alcohol Dependence. Official journal of the College on Problems of Drug Dependence. TOC, abstracts, order info, author guidelines. (http://www.elsevier.com/wps/find/journaldescription.cws_home/506052/description#description)

Drug and Alcohol Review. TOC, subscription information, instructions for contributors. (http://www.apsad.org.au/index.php?menu=drug)

Drug Dependence, Alcohol Abuse, and Alcoholism. Exerpta Medica Abstract Journal. Scope, order info. (http://www.elsevier.com/wps/find/journaldescription.cws_home/506008/description#description)

Drug Policy Analysis Bulletin. Newsletter of the Federation of American Scientists. (http://www.fas.org/drugs/)

Drugs: Education, Prevention & Policy. TOC, subscription information, instructions for contributors. (www.tandf.co.uk/journals/titles/09687637.html)

European Addiction Research. TOC, Author instructions, subscription information. (www.karger.com/ear)

International Journal of Drug Policy. Official journal of the International Harm Reduction Association. TOC, abstracts, order info, author guidelines. Full text of volumes 1 through 8 made available by DrugText. (http://www.sciencedi rect.com/science/journal/09553959)

International Journal of Drug Testing. Online journal, full text. (www.criminology.fsu.edu/journal)

Journal of Addiction and Mental Health. Centre for Addiction and Mental Health. Full text, order information. Published by Addiction Research Foundation. (www.camh.net)

Journal of Addictions Nursing. Official journal of the National Nurses Society on Addictions. Selected contents, instructions to authors, subscription information. (http://www.intnsa.org/jan.php)

Journal of Addictions and Offender Counseling. Official journal of the International Association of Addictions and Offender Counselors; author guidelines. (http://www.counseling.org/Publications/Journals.aspx) (http://www.accessmy library.com/coms2/browse_JJ_J172)

Journal of Addictive Diseases. Official journal of American Society on Addiction Medicine. TOC, abstracts, instructions for authors. (http://www.informa world.com/smpp/title~content=t792306884~db=all)

Journal of Alcohol and Drug Education. TOC, author guidelines. (http://www.uc.edu/healthpromotion/jade.html)

Journal of Alcohol and Drug Education. TOC, author guidelines. (www.unomaha.edu/~healthed/JADE.html)

Journal of Chemical Dependency Treatment. Official journal of the National Association of Addiction Treatment Professionals. TOC, subscription information, author guidelines. (http://www.informaworld.com/smpp/title~content=t904099375~db=all)

Journal of Child and Adolescent Substance Abuse. TOC, subscription information, author guidelines. (http://www.informaworld.com/smpp/title~content=t792303974~db=all)

Journal of Drug Education. Selected articles, author instructions, subscription information. (http://www.baywood.com/authors/ia/de.asp?id=0047–2379)

Journal of Drug Issues. TOC, author instructions, subscription information. (http://www2.criminology.fsu.edu/~jdi/)

Journal of Ethnicity in Substance Abuse (formerly *Drugs & Society*). TOC, subscription information, author guidelines. (http://www.informaworld.com/smpp/title~content=t792304000~db=all)

Journal of Maintenance in the Addictions. TOC, subscription information, author guidelines. (http://www.informaworld.com/smpp/title~db=all~content=t904 099607~tab=issueslist)

Journal of Ministry in Addiction and Recovery. TOC, subscription information, author guidelines. (http://www.informaworld.com/smpp/title~content=t9043 85076~db=all)

Journal of Psychoactive Drugs. (http://www.journalofpsychoactivedrugs.com/)

Journal of Social Work Practice in the Addictions. TOC, subscription information, author guidelines. (http://www.informaworld.com/smpp/title~content=t7923 06973~db=all)

Journal of Substance Abuse Treatment. TOC, author instructions, order information. (http://www.journalofsubstanceabusetreatment.com/)

Journal of Substance Use (formerly *Journal of Substance Misuse for Nursing, Health and Social Care*). TOC, scope. (http://www.informaworld.com/smpp/title~content=t713655978)

Journal of Workplace Behavioral Health (titled Employee Assistance Quarterly before 2004). TOC, subscription information, author instructions. (http://www.informaworld.com/smpp/title~db=all~content=t792306921~tab=issueslist)

Morbidity and Mortality Weekly Report (*MMWR*). Centers for Disease Control and Prevention publication. (www.cdc.gov/mmwr)

NIDA Notes. National Institute on Drug Abuse publication, full text. (www.drugabuse.gov/NIDA_Notes/NNIndex.html)

Prevention File: Alcohol, Tobacco, and Other Drugs. Subscription into, some issues full text. (http://www.silvergategroup.com/publications.htm)

Prevention Pipeline. Center for Substance Abuse Prevention (CSAP) publication. (www.health.org/pubs/prevpipe)

The Prevention Researcher. Newsletter published by Integrated Research Services. (www.health.org/govpubs/MS510/Articles.htm)

Psychology of Addictive Behaviors. Table of contents, abstracts, instructions for authors. (www.apa.org/journals/adb.html)

Pulse Check. U.S. Office of National Drug Control Policy publication index for this and other Office of National Drug Control Policy publications. (www.whitehousedrugpolicy.gov/publications/drugfact/pulsechk/f)

Self-Help Magazine. Full-text articles. (www.shpm.com)

Substance Abuse. Official journal of Association for Medical Education and Research in Substance Abuse. Editorial scope, subscription information (http://www.tandf.co.uk/journals/authors/WSUBauth.asp)

Substance Misuse Bulletin. Centre for Addiction Studies, London. (www.sghms.ac.uk/depts/addictive-behaviour/ infores/smb.htm)

Substance Use and Misuse. TOC with abstracts, author guidelines, order information. (http://www.informaworld.com/smpp/title~content=t713597302)

Information Sources and Databases

The following information including annotations that have been drawn from government publications and other resources in the public domain.

Center for Substance Abuse Treatment (CSAT), Substance Abuse and Mental Health Services Administration, U.S. Department of Health and Human Services. CSAT provides information about treatment improvement protocols, technical assistance publications, and other CSAT publications. (http://csat.samhsa.gov/)

ERIC. The world's largest source of education information, with more than 1 million abstracts of documents and journal articles on education research and practice. Coverage: 1966–present. (http://ericir.syr.edu/Eric)

Information on Drugs and Alcohol (IDA). IDA contains scientific literature relating to alcohol and substance abuse prevention and sociological literature. Provides abstracts and bibliographic records. (http://idasearch.health.org/compass)

Medline. PubMed, a service of the National Library of Medicine, provides access to more than 12 million Medline citations back to the mid-1960s and citations to additional life science journals. PubMed includes links to many sites providing full-text articles and other related resources. (www.ncbi.nlm.nih.gov/entrez/query.fcgi?db=PubMed)

MEDLINEplus. This is a source of good health information from the world's largest medical library, the National Library of Medicine. (http://www.nlm.nih.gov/medlineplus)

National Clearinghouse for Alcohol and Drug Information Prevline. Prevline is the database portal to the resources of the National Clearinghouse for Alcohol and Drug Information, the world's largest resource for current information and materials concerning substance abuse prevention. (http://ncadi.samhsa.gov/)

National Criminal Justice Reference Service (NCJRS). The NCJRS Abstracts Database contains summaries of more than 170,000 criminal justice publications, including federal, state, and local government reports, books, research reports, journal articles, and unpublished research. (http://www.ncjrs.gov/App/AbstractDB/AbstractDBSearch.aspx)

National Institute on Drug Abuse (NIDA) publications catalog. This semiannually updated catalog provides a listing of research monographs, clinical reports, surveys, brochures, prevention packets booklets, and posters. Videos are also available. (http://www.drugabuse.gov)

National Organization for the Reform of Marijuana Laws (NORML). NORML provides information resources about the right of adults to use marijuana responsibly, whether for medical or personal purposes. (http://www.norml.org)

National Substance Abuse Web Index (NSAWI). This search engine indexes 26 authoritative, public interest, and U.S. government Web sites for locating reliable information on prevention, treatment, alcohol, tobacco, and illicit drugs. NSAWI may be used to search through every document on prominent sites in the prevention world. Sites are re-indexed every two weeks. (http://nsawi.health.org)

PsycInfo. This is an abstract (not full-text) database of psychological literature from the 1800s to the present. More than a million records are available to search. (http://www.apa.org/psycinfo)

Schaffer Library of Drug Policy. The Schaffer Library is the largest Internet source addressing issues related to major studies of drugs and drug policy, history of drugs and drug laws, medical marijuana research, government publications on drugs and drug policy, charts and graphs of drug war statistics, and information on specific drugs. (http://www.druglibrary.org/schaffer/index.htm)

Substance Abuse Information Database (SAID). This database provides summaries and full texts of materials relating to workplace substance abuse issues. (http://www.dol.gov/asp/programs/drugs/said/)

Treatment Resource Database (TRD). The TRD provides bibliographic citations to alcohol and substance abuse treatment materials with a focus on intervention, recovery, treatment, and relapse prevention. (http://sadatabase.health.org/trd)

National Statistics

The following government sources provide information about multiple aspects of illicit drugs and related problems.

Bureau of Justice Statistics: Sourcebook of Criminal Justice Statistics Online. Data from more than 100 sources about all aspects of criminal justice in the United States. (http://www.albany.edu/sourcebook)

Federal Bureau of Investigation, Uniform Crime Reports.

National Center for Health Statistics (FASTSTATS). National health data and statistics. (http://www.cdc.gov/nchs/fastats/default.htm)

National Highway and Traffic Safety Administration, Fatality Analysis Reporting System (FARS). FARS contains data on all fatal traffic crashes within the 50 states, the District of Columbia, and Puerto Rico. (http://www-fars.nhtsa.dot.gov)

National Institute on Alcohol Abuse and Alcoholism (NIAAA)—Quick Facts. Provides tables presenting data on alcohol topics, including amounts and patterns of alcohol consumption, alcohol dependence or abuse, consequences of alcohol consumption, and other alcohol-related topics. (http://www.niaaa.nih.gov/Resources/DatabaseResources/QuickFacts/)

Statistics for crime in the United States. (http://www.fbi.gov/ucr/ucr.htm)

Substance Abuse and Mental Health Services Administration (SAMHSA), Office of Applied Studies (OAS). The most recent national data on alcohol, tobacco and other drugs from OAS surveys are found here. (http://www.oas.samhsa.gov/)

Web Sites

Web sites with good links to other substance abuse resources are marked with a double asterisk (**). The information presented on Web sites is drawn from material prepared by SALIS (http://salis.org/resources).

Alcohol, Tobacco, and Other Drugs (ATOD) Web Sites

Alcohol and Drug Abuse Institute Links, University of Washington** (http://depts.washington.edu/adai/links/links.htm)

European Gateway on Alcohol, Drugs, and Addiction (ELISAD Gateway), European Union (http://www.addictionsinfo.eu)

European Monitoring Centre for Drugs and Drug Addiction (EMCDDA), European Union (http://www.emcdda.europa.eu/)

Hazelden Foundation Resource Center** (http://www.hazelden.org/web/landing.view)

Health Web Substance Abuse, University of Minnesota Biomedical Library** (http://www.biomed.lib.umn.edu/help/guides/PUBH5003)

Minnesota Institute of Public Health Links** (http://www.miph.org/links.html)

Virtual Clearinghouse on Alcohol Tobacco and Other Drugs, International (English, French, Spanish)** (http://www.atod.org)

Web of Addictions** (http://www.well.com/user/woa)

General ATOD Web Sites

Centre for Addiction and Mental Health, Canada (http://www.camh.net)

Centre for Education and Information on Drugs and Alcohol, Australia (http://www.ceida.net.au)

Common Sense for Drug Policy, United States (http://www.csdp.org/)

Daily Dose, United Kingdom (http://dailydose.net)

DrugScope, United Kingdom (http://www.dsdaily.org.uk/)

Indiana Prevention Resource Center,** United States (http://www.drugs.indi ana.edu)

Join Together Online,** United States (http://www.jointogether.org)

National Clearinghouse for Alcohol and Drug Information—PREVLINE USA (http://ncadi.samhsa.gov/)

Regional Alcohol and Drug Awareness Resource—RADAR Network (SAMHSA), United States (http://ncadi.samhsa.gov/radar/)

SAMHSA Health Information Network, United States (http://www.samhsa.gov/shin/moreaboutshin.aspx)

Virtual Clearinghouse on Alcohol, Tobacco and Other Drugs,** Australia (http://www.atod.org)

Web of Addictions** (http://www.well.com/user/woa)

Government

European Monitoring Centre for Drugs and Drug Addiction (EMCDDA), European Union (http://www.emcdda.europa.eu/html.cfm/index190EN.html)

National Clearinghouse for Alcohol and Drug Information (NCADI) (http://ncadi.samhsa.gov/)

National Institute on Alcohol Abuse and Alcoholism (NIAAA) (http://www.niaaa.nih.gov/)

National Institute on Drug Abuse (NIDA) (http://www.nida.nih.gov)

Office of National Drug Control Policy (ONDCP) (http://www.whitehouse drugpolicy.gov)

Substance Abuse and Mental Health Services Administration (SAMHSA) (http://www.samhsa.gov)

United Nations International Drug Control Programme (http://www.unodc.org/)

United States Information Agency (USIA), Narcotics and Substance Abuse (http://usinfo.state.gov/topical/global/drugs)

Library Organizations

American Library Association (ALA), United States (http://www.ala.org)
Association of Mental Health Librarians, United States (http://www.mhlib.org)
European Association of Libraries and Information Services on Alcohol and Other Drugs (ELISAD), European Union (http://www.elisad.eu/)
Medical Library Association, Mental Health Special Interest Group, United States (http://www.miami.edu/mhsig)
Special Libraries Association (SLA), United States (http://www.sla.org)
Substance Abuse Librarians and Information Specialists (SALIS): An International Organization, United States (http://salis.org/resources/resources.html)

Policy-Related Organizations

Association for Medical education and Research in Substance Abuse (AMERSA), United States (http://www.amersa.org)
Canadian Centre on Substance Abuse, Canada** (http://www.ccsa.ca)
Drug Policy Alliance (formerly Lindesmith Center-Drug Policy Foundation),** United States (http://www.drugpolicy.org)
Marin Institute,** United States (http://www.marininstitute.org)
Office of National Drug Control Policy (ONDCP) (http://www.whitehouse drugpolicy.gov)

Research Institutes

Alcohol and Drug Abuse Institute, University of Washington** (http://depts.washington.edu/adai)
Alcohol Research Group, United States (http://www.arg.org)
Butler Center for Research (Hazelden), United States (http://www.hazelden.org/web/public/research.page)
Center for Alcohol and Addiction Studies, Brown University (http://www.caas.brown.edu/)
Center of Alcohol Studies, Rutgers University (http://alcoholstudies.rutgers.edu/)
Center for Substance Abuse Research, University of Maryland (http://www.cesar.umd.edu)
Centre for Addiction and Mental Health, Canada (http://www.camh.net)
Centre for Drug Research, University of Amsterdam (http://www.cedro-uva.org)
DrugScope, United Kingdom** (http://www.drugscope.org.uk)
Institute of Alcohol Studies, United Kingdom** (http://www.ias.org.uk)
Integrated Substance Abuse Programs (ISAP), University of California (http://www.uclaisap.org)
International Council on Alcohol, Drugs, and Traffic Safety, Norway (http://www.icadts.org/)
National Center on Addiction and Substance Abuse, Columbia University (http://www.casacolumbia.org)
Research Institute on Addictions, State University of New York at Buffalo (http://www.ria.buffalo.edu)

Special Topics

ATOD Serials Database, United States (http://lib.adai.washington.edu/salisserials.htm)
Higher Education Center for Alcohol and Other Drug Prevention, United States (http://www.higheredcenter.org/)
Historical Resources on Alcohol Use in America, Rutgers University (http://alcoholstudies.rutgers.edu/library/resources_files/comprehensive_resources/alcoholhistory_internet_all.html)
International Society of Addiction Journal Editors (http://www.parint.org/isajewebsite/index.htm)
Substance Abuse Screening & Assessment Instruments Database (http://lib.adai.washington.edu/instruments/)

Treatment

Alcoholics Anonymous, United States (http://www.aa.org/)
Hazelden Foundation,** United States (http://www.hazelden.org)
Narcotics Anonymous, United States (http://www.na.org)
Treatment Research Institute, United States (http://www.tresearch.org/)

Recommended Sites for Search and Information

The following Web sites are the personal recommendations of the authors for information on drug abuse topics.

Alcohol Problems and Solutions** (http://www2.potsdam.edu/hansondj/)
Campaign for Tobacco Free Kids** (http://tobaccofreekids.org)
Common Sense for Drug Policy** (http://www.csdp.org/)
Daily Dose** (http://dailydose.net/)
Google** (http://google.com)
Join Together Online** (http://www.jointogether.org)
Medline** (www.ncbi.nlm.nih.gov/entrez/query.fcgi?db=PubMed)
National Clearinghouse for Alcohol and Drug Information (NCADI)**
National Clearinghouse for Alcohol and Drug Information (NCADI)** Publications Catalog (http://www.health.gov)
Office of National Drug Control Policy (ONDCP)** (http://www.whitehouse drugpolicy.gov)
Schaffer Library of Drug Policy** (http://www.druglibrary.org/schaffer/index.htm)
Substance Abuse Librarians and Information Specialists (SALIS)** (http://salis.org/resources/resources.html)
Tips for Teens Publication Series** (http://www.health.gov)

INDEX

About the Authors

Richard E. Isralowitz, PhD, is professor and director of the Regional Alcohol and Drug Abuse Resources Center, Ben Gurion University. Dr. Isralowitz is author of numerous books and publications on drug use and abuse; he is a Fulbright Scholar and Distinguished International Scientist, National Institute on Drug Abuse.

Peter L. Myers, PhD, professor emeritus of addiction studies, is editor of the *Journal of Ethnicity in Substance Abuse* and past president of the International Coalition for Addiction Studies Education. Dr. Myers is author of numerous books and publications on drug abuse and abuse, and he coauthored the national standards for the accreditation of addiction curricula in higher education.